YOUR COMPLETE MEDICAL RECORD

BOOKS FROM THE
PEOPLE'S MEDICAL SOCIETY

Take This Book to the Hospital With You

How to Evaluate and Select a Nursing Home

Medicine on Trial

Medicare Made Easy

Your Medical Rights

Getting the Most for Your Medical Dollar

Take This Book to the Gynecologist With You

Take This Book to the Obstetrician With You

Healthy Body Book: Test Yourself for Maximum Health

Blood Pressure: Questions You Have . . . Answers You Need

Your Heart: Questions You Have . . . Answers You Need

The Consumer's Guide To Medical Lingo

150 Ways to Be a Savvy Medical Consumer

100 Ways to Live to 100

Take This Book to the Pediatrician With You

Dial 800 for Health

Arthritis: Questions You Have . . . Answers You Need

Diabetes: Questions You Have . . . Answers You Need

YOUR COMPLETE MEDICAL RECORD

Developed for the consumer by the

≡People's Medical Society

Allentown, Pennsylvania

The **People's Medical Society** is a nonprofit consumer health organization dedicated to the principles of better, more responsive and less expensive medical care. Organized in 1983, the People's Medical Society puts previously unavailable medical information into the hands of consumers so that they can make informed decisions about their own health care.

Membership in the People's Medical Society is $20 a year and includes a subscription to the *People's Medical Society Newsletter*. For information, write to the People's Medical Society, 462 Walnut Street, Allentown, PA 18102; or call (215) 770-1670.

This and other People's Medical Society publications are available for quantity purchase at discount. Contact the People's Medical Society for details.

CONTENTS

INTRODUCTION

Keeping your own and your family's medical record can be worthwhile, yet very few of us do it. We assume that the records our physicians, dentists, optometrists, and other practitioners keep are easy to obtain and completely accurate. Unfortunately, this is not always the case. Fewer than one-half of the states have specific laws guaranteeing consumers the right to their medical records. And many consumers who have received copies have found major discrepancies between their recollection of events and those noted in the records.

Since the founding of the People's Medical Society in 1983, we have received more mail from consumers complaining about access to, and quality of, their individual medical records than any single topic. Yet, upon inquiry, we found that virtually none of those who wrote to us had a system or even a file by which they kept track of their own conditions or encounters with the medical care system.

That is why we have put together this book. It is not designed as a substitute for the records that your medical practitioners should be maintaining. Rather, it is meant to serve as your own system of keeping tabs on your medical history and encounters. And by being as diligent as possible in keeping the records, you can work in true partnership with your medical care providers.

It is not unusual for a person to move numerous times during his or her lifetime, nor is it unusual for a person to encounter a dozen different doctors in the course of a few years. Compounding this fragmentation is the fact that doctors and hospitals do not keep track of what others of them have done for you. Too often, attempting to piece together the history of a medical event becomes a futile search through old bills and insurance records. But now, with this book, you can easily note and keep track of all your medical and health-related activities.

Each form in *Your Complete Medical Record* is designed for a specific purpose. The Family Medical History, for example, asks you to identify conditions or diseases that have affected members of your family. By doing this, you discover which relatives have or had conditions or diseases that may eventually affect your health or that may already have done so.

Women's health issues have not been overlooked in *Your Complete Medical Record.* Three specific forms address important women's health issues: the Family Obstetrical and Gynecological History, the Individual Gynecological Record, and the Prenatal Visits Record. The Family Obstetrical and Gynecologic History can be a valuable instrument for women interested in tracking familial conditions as far back as their grandmothers and as current as their siblings. The Individual Gynecological Record is used to keep track of all visits to gynecological practitioners. And the Prenatal Visits Record contains enough space to enter the results of each monthly obstetrical visit throughout a pregnancy—right up to the delivery.

Other forms permit you to track allergy problems, dental and vision care visits, prescription and nonprescription medications, diagnostic procedures, and hospitalizations. We have also included a form, Your Child's Medical Record, which recognizes that caring parents want to give their child a sound record of the child's medical history when he or she is older.

Getting Started

Each record includes specific instructions on how to complete the information requested. Some of your responses can be entered immediately, while others may require a review of old family records just to make sure that Grandma or Grandpa actually had a certain condition.

After you provide the preliminary information, use each record as needed or when appropriate. For instance, when you see a medical provider, have a prescription filled, or require a diagnostic procedure, enter the information on the proper chart. Enter as much or as little information as you see fit; after all, it's your medical record. Just remember that the more complete your entries, the better these records can serve you.

Keeping and maintaining a personal medical record is not difficult. It is the mark of an informed and educated medical consumer.

Accessing Your Medical Records

State Laws

Requesting and receiving copies of your medical records from doctors, dentists, chiropractors, hospitals, or mental health facilities should be a relatively easy process, yet most consumers find it a struggle. Since laws governing access to medical records are enacted at the state level, what has emerged is a patchwork of confusing laws, court decisions, and health department regulations that make the process anything but clear and easy.

Only 24 states have some form of legislation that permits you direct access to your medical records. These states are:

Alaska	Minnesota
Arkansas	Montana
California	Nevada
Colorado	New Hampshire
Connecticut	New Jersey
Florida	New York
Georgia	Oklahoma
Hawaii	South Dakota
Indiana	Virginia
Louisiana	Washington
Maryland	West Virginia
Michigan	Wisconsin

Physicians in Maine, Massachusetts, and Texas have the option of providing you with a summary of your records if they choose not to release your entire record. If you did not find your state listed here, then there are no regulations governing consumer access to copies of medical records.

Don't despair! Even if your state has no regulation covering your direct access to your medical records, there is nothing to preclude your asking a practitioner or facility for copies of your records. In fact, we encourage you to do so.

As with any administrative request, knowing the formalities and going about the request in the proper way help guarantee the best outcome. We recommend you use the following procedure.

1) Contact the practitioner or facility that has your records and ask about their general procedures for releasing records. Take notes on what is said and ask additional questions if the process seems confusing. If your state is one of those with access laws, let the contact person at the office or the facility know that you know your rights of access. Some office managers and other clerical personnel often claim that it is illegal for you to have copies of your records. When this happens, ask what specific state law prohibits access. Re-

member, there is no state where it is illegal to obtain copies of your medical record.

2) Always put your request in writing. This documents your efforts and is proof that you are working through normal channels. Include your name, address, patient identification number (if known), and the specific entry or file that you want. Indicate your willingness to pay reasonable copying fees (we consider unreasonable anything over $.50 a page).

3) If your initial request is denied by the office manager or records administrator, ask her to put the denial in writing. Also ask her to cite the reasons you are being denied access to your records—for example, state law, health department regulation, or office policy. Then ask her to cite the statute number or specific regulation.

4) Learn about any appeals process that permits you to resubmit your request for specific parts of your record.

5) Contact the hospital patient representative if you are having problems obtaining hospital records. You may wish to consider asking a physician-ally to request copies of your records.

6) When all else fails, contact a lawyer familiar with your state's laws. You may be able to obtain a court order from a magistrate or civil court judge if you can show good cause for needing your medical records.

Federal Laws

Access to your medical records from federal hospitals—including military, Veterans Administration, and prison hospitals—is covered under the federal Privacy Act and the Freedom of Information Act. A person still in active duty must write to the hospital at his post or at the previous duty station. Retirees and anyone else no longer in active duty must write the National Archives Record Center, 9700 Page, St. Louis, MO 63132. Be sure to include your military identification number, branch of service, and dates of service.

Medical Information Bureau

You may never have heard of the Medical Information Bureau (MIB), but it has heard of you. In fact, it probably knows more about you and your health than you can imagine. How is this possible, you ask? If you have ever completed an insurance company application form, you know that these companies want to know a lot about your present and past medical history. And most people comply and answer the many detailed questions. The chances are excellent that the information you provided on the application found its way to the MIB.

Because insurance companies rely upon the information stored at the MIB to determine whether or not they will insure you, it is very important that your file is accurate. Unfortunately, your right to inspect your file is limited to all nonmedical information, the names of insurance companies that reported information to the MIB, and the names of insurance companies that received a copy of the information in your file within the last six months preceding your request.

The MIB discloses medical information to physicians. Ask your physician to assist you in obtaining the medical information contained in your file. Write to the MIB and ask for a copy of the form "Request for Disclosure of MIB Record Information":

Medical Information Bureau
P.O. Box 105, Essex Station
Boston, MA 02112
(617) 329-4500

QUICK REFERENCE GUIDE

The first step in being prepared for a medical emergency is to have the names of important groups and their telephone numbers at your fingertips. This Quick Reference Guide eliminates the need to flip through a telephone directory to find important numbers. Being able to quickly locate an emergency telephone number could mean the difference between life and death.

Begin by listing ambulance companies that serve your area and/or those to which you belong. Some communities continue to operate ambulance squads as part of their public safety departments. Make sure you include the correct telephone number, especially if your area is not served by a 911 emergency telephone system. Incorrectly dialing 911 when the service is not available in your calling area could result in a potentially harmful delay.

Crisis hotlines—operated, for example, by self-help groups for substance abuse or domestic violence—can be a source of information and reassurance. They may also be able to refer you to other organizations and agencies in your community. We suggest that you begin by listing all local crisis hotlines, then regional, followed by national hotlines.

List the pharmacies you use. Be aware, however, that it's a good practice to use one pharmacy for all your prescription drugs since your medication record is complete at that one location. Unless all medications are noted on one profile, you and your pharmacist cannot monitor potential drug interactions.

Even if you don't have children or pets—but especially if you do—your local poison control center should be listed here. Poison control centers provide both emergency and general information about poisons and other substances that could have poisonous effects on the body.

Always keep the Quick Reference Guide up-to-date. Don't run the risk of needing to contact a particular group in an emergency, only to find that the number has been disconnected or changed. At least once a year, check all the numbers on this chart. The best way to do this? Call the numbers one by one.

QUICK REFERENCE GUIDE

Use this chart to list emergency telephone numbers and the telephone numbers of your various practitioners and other frequently called medical services.

Organization	Address	Telephone
Ambulance Service		
Crisis Hotlines		
Poison Control Center		
Police/Fire		

Doctors and other practitioners		
Name	Specialty	Telephone

QUICK REFERENCE GUIDE

Hospital	Address	Telephone

Pharmacy	Address	Telephone

ADDITIONAL TELEPHONE NUMBERS

Organizations	Telephone

FAMILY MEDICAL HISTORY

Completing the Family Medical History can be relatively easy if you carefully review the list of conditions or diseases prior to entering any information. In the first column is a list of the most common conditions or diseases, ranging from allergies to vertigo. Some of the conditions, such as digestive diseases, have more than one choice since there are various diseases that fall into this category. The chart is further divided into three columns for family members: grandparents, parents, and siblings.

These examples illustrate how to compile your family medical history: If, for example, your paternal grandfather had osteoarthritis, you would place a check mark in the column "Grandparents, Paternal." If your mother has diabetes, indicate such in the appropriate column under the heading "Parents, Mother." Do the same for all your siblings. Also enter the age at onset in the same column.

Since there is a good chance you do not know everything—or perhaps even much—about your family's medical history, you should check with other family members for additional information. Don't be surprised, however, if you can't obtain all the information you require. Some people may be reluctant to discuss certain conditions, because at one time it was considered rude to know other family members' health problems. We suggest you do the best you can, especially with your parents and siblings.

Use Part 2 of the medical history to elaborate on any condition or to list a condition or disease not found on the chart. Enter the family member's name and relationship, the condition or disease, and any other information you believe is relevant to a family medical history.

FAMILY MEDICAL HISTORY

Part 1

In Part 1 indicate by check mark those conditions or diseases a particular family member has or had. Also note the family member's age at onset of the disease.

Condition/Disease	Grandparents		Parents		Siblings			
	Maternal	Paternal	Mother	Father				
Allergies								
Animals								
Foods								
Grasses								
Insect bites/stings								
Medications								
Molds								
Pollens								
Synthetic/ Manufactured products								
Others								
Alzheimer's								
Arthritis								
Infectious								
Juvenile RA								
Osteoarthritis								
Rheumatoid								
Asthma								
Blood disorders								
Anemia								
Hemophilia (abnormal bleeding)								
Thrombosis (abnormal clotting)								
Bone fractures								
Skull								
Neck								
Collar								
Shoulder								
Arm								
Wrist								
Hand								
Finger								

Part 1 (Continued)

Condition/Disease	Grandparents		Parents		Siblings			
	Maternal	Paternal	Mother	Father				
Rib								
Spine								
Pelvis								
Hip								
Leg								
Knee								
Ankle								
Foot								
Toe								
Cancer								
Basal cell carcinoma (skin)								
Bladder								
Bone								
Breast								
Cervix								
Colon and rectum								
Leukemia								
Liver								
Lungs								
Lymphoma								
Malignant melanoma (skin)								
Oral (mouth and gums)								
Ovarian								
Pancreas								
Prostate								
Squamous cell carcinoma (skin)								
Stomach								
Testicles								
Throat								
Uterus								
Coronary artery and heart diseases								
Angina								
Arrhythmia (abnormal heartbeat)								
Arteriosclerosis (hardening of the arteries)								
Atherosclerosis (fatty deposits on artery walls)								

Part 1 (Continued)

Condition/Disease	Grandparents		Parents		Siblings			
	Maternal	Paternal	Mother	Father				
Congenital defect (present at birth)								
Congestive heart failure								
Endocarditis (infection around the heart)								
Enlarged heart								
Heart valve problems (aortic, mitral, pulmonary, tricuspid)								
Myocardial infarction (heart attack)								
Diabetes								
type I								
type II								
Digestive diseases								
Crohn's disease								
Diverticulitis								
Duodenal ulcer								
Duodenitis (inflammation of the duodenum)								
Gallstones								
Hiatal hernia								
Ulcerative colitis								
Eating disorders								
Anorexia								
Bulimia								
Epilepsy								
Eye conditions								
Cataracts								
Diabetic retinopathy								
Glaucoma								
Macular degeneration								
Retinal detachment								
Gout								
Headache								
Cluster								
Migraine								
Sinus								
Tension								
Other								

Part 1 (Continued)

Condition/Disease	Grandparents		Parents		Siblings			
	Maternal	Paternal	Mother	Father				
Head injury								
Concussion								
Fracture								
Hearing disorders								
Infection								
Loss of hearing								
Nerve damage								
Punctured eardrum								
Tinnitus (ringing)								
Hernia								
Epigastric								
Femoral								
Incisional								
Inguinal								
Umbilical								
Hypertension (high blood pressure)								
Hypotension (abnormally low blood pressure)								
Incontinence								
Bladder								
Bowel								
Kidney diseases								
Infection								
Stones								
Tumors								
Liver diseases								
Cirrhosis								
Enlarged liver								
Hemochromatosis (excess iron in the liver)								
Hepatitis A								
Hepatitis B								
Non-A/Non-B Hepatitis								
Tumors								
Lung diseases								
Asbestosis ("white lung")								
Asthma								

Part 1 (Continued)

Condition/Disease	Grandparents		Parents		Siblings			
	Maternal	Paternal	Mother	Father				
Bronchitis								
Byssinosis ("brown lung")								
Pleurisy								
Pneumoconiosis ("black lung")								
Pneumonia								
Tuberculosis								
Tumors								
Lupus								
Mental illnesses								
Osteoporosis								
Parkinson's disease								
Sexually transmitted diseases								
AIDS								
Chlamydia								
Genital warts								
Gonorrhea								
Herpes								
HIV								
Syphilis								
Skin conditions								
Eczema								
Moles								
Psoriasis								
Tumors								
Warts								
Others								
Stroke								
Vertigo (dizziness)								

FAMILY MEDICAL HISTORY

Part 2

Use this page to record additional information or comments concerning any condition or disease experienced by family members.

Condition/Disease	Family Member	Comments

Part 2 (Continued)

Condition/Disease	Family Member	Comments

FAMILY OBSTETRICAL AND GYNECOLOGICAL HISTORY

Knowing the obstetrical and gynecological history of your family can help you track any conditions or problems that may have an effect on your own health.

Use the first part to record the obstetrical and gynecological conditions or problems experienced by your grandmother, mother, female siblings, and other female relatives. (Regarding the latter, we suggest you list only those who are biologically related, such as cousins and aunts.) List the names of your female siblings and other female relatives in the spaces provided. Carefully examine each condition and indicate by a check mark those relatives who experienced such problems. Also enter age at onset in the same column. So that the record is as accurate as it can be, you may need to consult with family members to ensure that you have all your facts straight— or that you have any facts at all.

In Part 2 list additional comments concerning any condition or problem experienced by a female relative. The conditions enumerated in Part 1 are merely some of the most common and are not meant to comprise an entire list of possibilities.

Remember, the purpose of constructing this family history is to alert you to potential health problems that you could face. For example, cervical cancer, one of the most deadly forms of female cancers, can run in families. The normal risk of this disease is about one woman in 70, or 1.4 percent; however, if two or more first-degree relatives have it, your risk jumps to 50 percent. Breast cancer is another good example. Its incidence is about one woman in nine, or 11 percent. In addition, researchers have discovered that if your mother, grandmothers, or sisters developed breast cancer before age 45 or in both breasts, your risk for developing breast cancer is higher than normal. In either of these examples, foreknowledge, combined with early screening and detection, may mean the difference between life and death.

FAMILY OBSTETRICAL AND GYNECOLOGICAL HISTORY

Part 1

In Part 1 indicate by a check mark those conditions or problems experienced by your grandmothers, mother, female sibling(s), and other immediate female relatives (including biological aunts). Also indicate age at onset, if known.

Condition/Problem	Grandmothers	Mother	Female sibling(s) and other female family members		
Abnormal breast exam					
Abnormal Pap smear					
Abnormal pelvic exam					
Abortion (elective)					
Age began menstruating					
Average # of days in cycle					
Average length of period					
Birth control pills					
Bleeding between periods					
Breast biopsy					
Cervical biopsy					
Colposcopy					
DES (diethylstilbestrol) exposure					
Endometrial biopsy					
Fragile bones					
Hormone replacement therapy					
IUD					
Menopause					
Miscarriage					
Painful breasts					
Painful intercourse					
Painful menstruation					
Pregnancies					
Premenstrual symptoms					
Sexual dissatisfaction					
Sexually transmitted diseases					
Tubal ligation					
Tumors—breasts					
Tumors—ovaries					
Tumors—uterus					
Vaginal infections					
Others					

FAMILY OBSTETRICAL AND GYNECOLOGICAL HISTORY

Part 2

List additional information or comments concerning any condition or problem experienced by a female family member. This section may also be used to list any condition or problem not covered in Part 1.

Name of Family Member	Relationship	Condition/Problem	Age at Onset

Part 2 (Continued)

Name of Family Member	Relationship	Condition/Problem	Age at Onset

PERSONAL MEDICAL HISTORY

If you have already recorded the information called for in the Family Medical History, completing your own medical history should not be difficult. Part 1 requests current personal data, as well as information about your birth. You may need to have a copy of your birth certificate handy in order to complete some of the questions. Obviously, your parents, other relatives, and the hospital in which you were born are more sources of information.

Part 2 asks you to indicate those conditions or diseases that you have or had and your age at onset. This section is similar to the one found in the Family Medical History, except for the addition of illnesses you most likely had in early childhood. You may need to obtain copies of your pediatric record from your pediatrician or family doctor if you can't recall the details requested. If either physician is no longer in practice, try getting in touch with his or her successor to determine if the old records have been put in storage or are still available. The next best source of old records is the hospital where your pediatrician or family doctor had admitting privileges. (See "Accessing Your Medical Records," page 8.)

In Part 3 enter all immunizations, or vaccinations, you received in childhood and throughout adulthood. To help you get started, we've listed the most common ones. Don't forget, however, to list other immunizations you may have had for special situations: for example, vaccinations for plague, typhoid, yellow fever, cholera, and so on. Much of the information you require is probably contained in your early childhood medical records; therefore, it's a good idea to contact as many of your former childhood doctors as possible so you can have a complete record of immunizations.

Equally important to note are any side effects or adverse reactions you experience or experienced as a result of an immunization. If you later develop a condition that has been found to be linked to a specific vaccine, you can verify whether you did or did not have that vaccination.

PERSONAL MEDICAL HISTORY

Part 1
Personal Data

Enter the personal information as requested to complete Part 1 of your record.

Name			
Address			
City		St	Zip
Telephone (home)		(work)	
In case of emergency, notify			
Relationship	Telephone (home)		(work)
Date of birth	Time of birth	A.M	P.M.
Weight lbs oz	Length inches		
Blood type	APGAR score	PKU test	
Place of birth			
City		St	
Hospital			
Address			
Birthing center			
Address			
Other			
Vaginal birth ☐ Yes ☐ No	C-section ☐ Yes☐ No		
Full term ☐ Yes☐ No If no, how many weeks premature			

List any birthmark, birth defect, or complication noted at birth. List any distinguishing mark you have, including scars (natural or surgical).

_____

_____

_____

_____

_____

_____

_____

Attending physician
Nurse-midwife
Other practitioner

Part 2
Conditions List

Indicate by check mark those conditions or diseases that you have or had, including age at onset.

Condition	Age	Condition	Age
Allergies		Knee	
Animals		Ankle	
Foods		Foot	
Grasses		Toe	
Insect bites/stings		Cancer	
Medications		Basal cell carcinoma (skin)	
Molds		Bladder	
Pollens		Bone	
Synthetic/Manufactured		Breast	
products		Cervix	
Others		Colon and rectum	
		Leukemia	
Arthritis		Liver	
Infectious		Lungs	
Juvenile RA		Lymphoma	
Osteoarthritis		Malignant melanoma (skin)	
Rheumatoid		Oral (mouth and gums)	
Asthma		Ovarian	
Blood disorders		Pancreas	
Anemia		Prostate	
Hemophilia (abnormal bleeding)		Squamous cell carcinoma (skin)	
Thrombosis (abnormal clotting)		Stomach	
Bone fractures		Testicles	
Skull		Throat	
Neck		Uterus	
Finger		Chicken pox	
Hand		Coronary artery and	
Wrist		heart diseases	
Arm		Angina	
Shoulder		Arrhythmia (abnormal heartbeat)	
Collar		Arteriosclerosis (hardening of	
Rib		the arteries)	
Spine		Atherosclerosis (fatty deposits	
Pelvis		on artery walls)	
Hip		Congenital defect (present at birth)	
Leg		Congestive heart failure	

Part 2 (Continued)
Conditions List

Condition	Age	Condition	Age
Endocarditis		Sinus	
Enlarged heart		Tension	
Heart valve problems (aortic, mitral, pulmonary, tricuspid)		Other	
Myocardial Infarction (heart attack)		Head Injuries	
Diabetes		Concussion	
type I		Fracture	
type II		Hearing disorders	
Digestive Diseases		Loss of hearing	
Blood in stools		Nerve damage	
Crohn's disease		Otitis media (middle ear infection)	
Duodenal ulcer		Punctured eardrum	
Duodenitis (inflammation of the duodenum)		Tinnitus (ringing)	
Diverticulitis		Hemorrhoids	
Gallstones		Hernia	
Hiatal hernia		Epigastric	
Tarry stools		Femoral	
Ulcerative colitis		Incisional	
Diphtheria		Inguinal	
Eating Disorders		Umbilical	
Anorexia		Hypertension (high blood pressure)	
Bulimia		Incontinence	
Epilepsy		Bladder	
Eye and vision conditions		Bowel	
Amblyopia (lazy eye)		Kidney diseases	
Astigmatism		Infection	
Cataracts		Stones	
Conjunctivitis		Tumors	
Glaucoma		Liver diseases	
Hyperopia (farsightedness)		Cirrhosis	
Macular degeneration		Enlarged liver	
Myopia (nearsightedness)		Hemochromatosis	
Retinal detachment		Hepatitis A	
Strabismus (misaligned eyes)		Hepatitis B	
Gout		Non-A/Non-B Hepatitis	
Headache		Tumors	
Cluster		Lung diseases	
Migraine		Asbestosis ("white lung")	
		Asthma	

Part 2 (Continued)
Conditions List

Condition	Age	Condition	Age
Bronchitis		Skin conditions	
Byssinosis ("brown lung")		Acne	
Chronic cough		Athlete's foot	
Emphysema		Birthmarks	
Pleurisy		Eczema	
Pneumoconiosis ("black lung")		Moles	
Pneumonia		Psoriasis	
Tuberculosis		Rash	
Lupus		Tumors	
Measles		Warts	
Meningitis		Other	
Mental illness		Stroke	
Mononucleosis		Tetanus	
Mumps		Typhoid fever	
Nervous system disorders		Urinary tract conditions	
Fainting		Bladder infections	
Memory loss		Bladder stones	
Muscle weakness		Blocked ureter	
Neuralgia		Excessive urination	
Numbness in limbs		Painful urination	
Seizures		Varicose veins	
Osteoporosis		Vertigo (dizziness)	
Parkinson's disease			
Pertussis (whooping cough)			
Polio			
Prostate disorders			
Rheumatic fever			
Rubella (German measles)			
Scarlet fever			
Sexual dysfunctions			
Sexually transmitted diseases			
AIDS			
Chlamydia			
Genital warts			
Gonorrhea			
Herpes			
HIV			
Syphilis			
Shingles			

Part 2 (Continued)
Conditions List

Use this page to record additional information concerning any of the conditions or diseases you checked in Part 2.

Condition	Age	Comment

Part 2 (Continued)
Conditions List

Condition	Age	Comment

Part 3
Immunizations History

Include all immunizations (vaccinations) you had from birth to the present and any side effects (unwanted effects, such as dizziness, headache, or dry mouth) or adverse reactions (harmful, potentially life-threatening effects, such as anaphylactic shock, cardiac arrhythmia, or irregular breathing) you experience or have experienced.

Vaccine	Date	Age	Physician/ Nurse	Side effects or adverse reactions experienced
Diphtheria, pertussis, tetanus (DPT)				
Oral polio vaccine				
Haemophilus influenzae type b (Hib)				
Hepatitis B (HBV)				
Measles, mumps, rubella (MMR)				
Tetanus and diphtheria (Td)				
Smallpox				

ALLERGY SYMPTOMS AND TREATMENT RECORD

The Allergy Symptoms and Treatment Record is used to record any type of allergic symptom that you experience. You can also use it as an ongoing record of all the treatments you receive for allergic conditions. In Part 1 enter the name of your allergist and/or any other medical practitioner you see for such problems. Here, too, you should summarize your known allergies. To help you, we've listed some of the most common ones.

Part 2 is the place to record the symptoms that you experience and suspect could be allergy-related. Always enter the date when you experience any such symptoms. This helps you establish a pattern of symptoms and may give you a clue as to their cause. Next, describe in detail your symptoms, using such words as *sneezing, coughing, swelling, watery eyes, puffiness, itching,* and so on. Your accuracy in describing symptoms will aid your allergist or other practitioner in diagnosing your problem.

In the "Tests and Diagnosis" column, record all specific tests ordered by your doctor. For example, initial testing may include the skin prick test (in which various substances are tested directly on your skin) or the radioallergosorbent, or RAST, test (a blood test that measures the amount of allergen that is circulating in your blood). Other tests may follow, such as a sinus X ray and a double-blind food allergy test. If you're unsure of the name of the test or procedure being ordered, ask your practitioner for an explanation. Next, enter the diagnosis.

Use the "Treatment" column to list all medications (including injections) given during each visit. If you're on a regular schedule of allergy treatments, make sure you record the date and type of injections you receive. Also record any therapeutic instructions you are given, such as avoidance of certain products or foods.

If properly maintained and detailed, this record can be of great value to anyone attempting to trace the progression of allergic symptoms and determine their cause. Be sure to make additional copies of the "Allergic Symptoms and Treatment" page. And remember to keep all copies in this record so you'll have them when needed.

ALLERGY SYMPTOMS AND TREATMENT RECORD

Part 1
Personal Data

Allergist _____

Address _____ Suite _____

City _____ St _____ Zip _____

Telephone _____

Physician _____

Address _____ Suite _____

City _____ St _____ Zip _____

Telephone _____

Known or suspected allergies: ☐ Animals ☐ Foods ☐ Grasses ☐ Molds
☐ Pollens ☐ Insect bites/stings ☐ Synthetic/Manufactured products
☐ Others _____

Part 2
Symptoms and Treatments

Enter the date you experience any symptoms that you believe
could be allergy-related. Describe your symptoms in terms such
as *sneezing, coughing, itching, watery eyes, swelling*, and so on.
Also list all diagnostic tests ordered by your allergist, results
of the tests, medications administered or prescribed, and any
special instructions you receive relating to diet, exercise or
life-style.

Date	Symptoms	Tests and Diagnosis	Treatment

ALLERGY SYMPTOMS AND TREATMENT RECORD

Date	Symptoms	Tests and Diagnosis	Treatment

ALLERGY SYMPTOMS AND TREATMENT RECORD

Date	Symptoms	Tests and Diagnosis	Treatment

BLOOD PRESSURE—CHOLESTEROL LEVELS—WEIGHT RECORD

Keeping track of your blood pressure, cholesterol levels, and weight is a very important aspect of being an informed and responsible—not to mention healthy—consumer. It's relatively easy to monitor your own blood pressure and weight since self-measuring devices (blood pressure cuffs and scales) are readily available. You should also record all measurements made by any medical practitioner. Cholesterol testing, however, usually involves an order from your physician and a trip to a laboratory.

In the first column enter the date your blood pressure, cholesterol levels, and/or weight is taken. When recording your blood pressure—which is the force of your blood's trip from your heart to and through the rest of your arterial and vascular system—be sure to enter both the systolic and diastolic readings. We've provided a slanted line in the second column to make it easier to record the two readings: for example, 120/80 (expressed as "120 over 80") or 150/95, and so on. The first number is the systolic, and the second number is the diastolic. Your practitioner can give you information on what is considered normal or high blood pressure.

Cholesterol levels are determined by a blood test, which means you'll be making a trip to a laboratory to have blood drawn for the test. When you return to your practitioner for the lab report or when it is sent to you, your cholesterol level will contain three separate numbers. One is the low-density lipoprotein, or LDL—called the "bad" cholesterol—which is the major contributor to clogged arteries. The other is high-density lipoprotein, or HDL—called the "good" cholesterol—which is thought to be a protective factor against heart disease. The combination of your LDL and HDL is your total cholesterol reading. Enter all three numbers in the space provided.

Enter your weight in the appropriate column every time you or your medical practitioner measures it. Keeping an accurate record of your weight can be helpful, especially if you're dieting and want to track your weight loss.

BLOOD PRESSURE – CHOLESTEROL LEVELS – WEIGHT RECORD

Enter your blood pressure, cholesterol levels, and weight each time you have them checked by a physician, nurse, or medical technician. Also enter all self-administered readings you take with monitoring devices, such as a blood pressure cuff or bathroom scale. (BP means blood pressure. WT means weight.)

Date	BP	Cholesterol	WT	Date	BP	Cholesterol	WT
		LDL___ HDL___ Total____				LDL___ HDL___ Total____	
		LDL___ HDL___ Total____				LDL___ HDL___ Total____	
		LDL___ HDL___ Total____				LDL___ HDL___ Total____	
		LDL___ HDL___ Total____				LDL___ HDL___ Total____	
		LDL___ HDL___ Total____				LDL___ HDL___ Total____	
		LDL___ HDL___ Total____				LDL___ HDL___ Total____	
		LDL___ HDL___ Total____				LDL___ HDL___ Total____	
		LDL___ HDL___ Total____				LDL___ HDL___ Total____	
		LDL___ HDL___ Total____				LDL___ HDL___ Total____	
		LDL___ HDL___ Total____				LDL___ HDL___ Total____	
		LDL___ HDL___ Total____				LDL___ HDL___ Total____	
		LDL___ HDL___ Total____				LDL___ HDL___ Total____	
		LDL___ HDL___ Total____				LDL___ HDL___ Total____	
		LDL___ HDL___ Total____				LDL___ HDL___ Total____	
		LDL___ HDL___ Total____				LDL___ HDL___ Total____	
		LDL___ HDL___ Total____				LDL___ HDL___ Total____	
		LDL___ HDL___ Total____				LDL___ HDL___ Total____	
		LDL___ HDL___ Total____				LDL___ HDL___ Total____	

BLOOD PRESSURE – CHOLESTEROL LEVELS – WEIGHT RECORD

Date	BP	Cholesterol	WT	Date	BP	Cholesterol	WT
		LDL___ HDL___ Total____				LDL___ HDL___ Total____	
		LDL___ HDL___ Total____				LDL___ HDL___ Total____	
		LDL___ HDL___ Total____				LDL___ HDL___ Total____	
		LDL___ HDL___ Total____				LDL___ HDL___ Total____	
		LDL___ HDL___ Total____				LDL___ HDL___ Total____	
		LDL___ HDL___ Total____				LDL___ HDL___ Total____	
		LDL___ HDL___ Total____				LDL___ HDL___ Total____	
		LDL___ HDL___ Total____				LDL___ HDL___ Total____	
		LDL___ HDL___ Total____				LDL___ HDL___ Total____	
		LDL___ HDL___ Total____				LDL___ HDL___ Total____	
		LDL___ HDL___ Total____				LDL___ HDL___ Total____	
		LDL___ HDL___ Total____				LDL___ HDL___ Total____	
		LDL___ HDL___ Total____				LDL___ HDL___ Total____	
		LDL___ HDL___ Total____				LDL___ HDL___ Total____	
		LDL___ HDL___ Total____				LDL___ HDL___ Total____	
		LDL___ HDL___ Total____				LDL___ HDL___ Total____	
		LDL___ HDL___ Total____				LDL___ HDL___ Total____	
		LDL___ HDL___ Total____				LDL___ HDL___ Total____	
		LDL___ HDL___ Total____				LDL___ HDL___ Total____	
		LDL___ HDL___ Total____				LDL___ HDL___ Total____	

BLOOD PRESSURE – CHOLESTEROL LEVELS – WEIGHT RECORD

Date	BP	Cholesterol	WT	Date	BP	Cholesterol	WT
		LDL___ HDL___ Total____				LDL___ HDL___ Total____	
		LDL___ HDL___ Total____				LDL___ HDL___ Total____	
		LDL___ HDL___ Total____				LDL___ HDL___ Total____	
		LDL___ HDL___ Total____				LDL___ HDL___ Total____	
		LDL___ HDL___ Total____				LDL___ HDL___ Total____	
		LDL___ HDL___ Total____				LDL___ HDL___ Total____	
		LDL___ HDL___ Total____				LDL___ HDL___ Total____	
		LDL___ HDL___ Total____				LDL___ HDL___ Total____	
		LDL___ HDL___ Total____				LDL___ HDL___ Total____	
		LDL___ HDL___ Total____				LDL___ HDL___ Total____	
		LDL___ HDL___ Total____				LDL___ HDL___ Total____	
		LDL___ HDL___ Total____				LDL___ HDL___ Total____	
		LDL___ HDL___ Total____				LDL___ HDL___ Total____	
		LDL___ HDL___ Total____				LDL___ HDL___ Total____	
		LDL___ HDL___ Total____				LDL___ HDL___ Total____	
		LDL___ HDL___ Total____				LDL___ HDL___ Total____	
		LDL___ HDL___ Total____				LDL___ HDL___ Total____	
		LDL___ HDL___ Total____				LDL___ HDL___ Total____	
		LDL___ HDL___ Total____				LDL___ HDL___ Total____	
		LDL___ HDL___ Total____				LDL___ HDL___ Total____	
		LDL___ HDL___ Total____				LDL___ HDL___ Total____	

BLOOD PRESSURE – CHOLESTEROL LEVELS – WEIGHT RECORD

Date	BP	Cholesterol	WT	Date	BP	Cholesterol	WT
		LDL___ HDL___ Total____				LDL___ HDL___ Total____	
		LDL___ HDL___ Total____				LDL___ HDL___ Total____	
		LDL___ HDL___ Total____				LDL___ HDL___ Total____	
		LDL___ HDL___ Total____				LDL___ HDL___ Total____	
		LDL___ HDL___ Total____				LDL___ HDL___ Total____	
		LDL___ HDL___ Total____				LDL___ HDL___ Total____	
		LDL___ HDL___ Total____				LDL___ HDL___ Total____	
		LDL___ HDL___ Total____				LDL___ HDL___ Total____	
		LDL___ HDL___ Total____				LDL___ HDL___ Total____	
		LDL___ HDL___ Total____				LDL___ HDL___ Total____	
		LDL___ HDL___ Total____				LDL___ HDL___ Total____	
		LDL___ HDL___ Total____				LDL___ HDL___ Total____	
		LDL___ HDL___ Total____				LDL___ HDL___ Total____	
		LDL___ HDL___ Total____				LDL___ HDL___ Total____	
		LDL___ HDL___ Total____				LDL___ HDL___ Total____	
		LDL___ HDL___ Total____				LDL___ HDL___ Total____	
		LDL___ HDL___ Total____				LDL___ HDL___ Total____	
		LDL___ HDL___ Total____				LDL___ HDL___ Total____	
		LDL___ HDL___ Total____				LDL___ HDL___ Total____	
		LDL___ HDL___ Total____				LDL___ HDL___ Total____	
		LDL___ HDL___ Total____				LDL___ HDL___ Total____	

BLOOD PRESSURE – CHOLESTEROL LEVELS – WEIGHT RECORD

Date	BP	Cholesterol	WT	Date	BP	Cholesterol	WT
		LDL___ HDL___ Total____				LDL___ HDL___ Total____	
		LDL___ HDL___ Total____				LDL___ HDL___ Total____	
		LDL___ HDL___ Total____				LDL___ HDL___ Total____	
		LDL___ HDL___ Total____				LDL___ HDL___ Total____	
		LDL___ HDL___ Total____				LDL___ HDL___ Total____	
		LDL___ HDL___ Total____				LDL___ HDL___ Total____	
		LDL___ HDL___ Total____				LDL___ HDL___ Total____	
		LDL___ HDL___ Total____				LDL___ HDL___ Total____	
		LDL___ HDL___ Total____				LDL___ HDL___ Total____	
		LDL___ HDL___ Total____				LDL___ HDL___ Total____	
		LDL___ HDL___ Total____				LDL___ HDL___ Total____	
		LDL___ HDL___ Total____				LDL___ HDL___ Total____	
		LDL___ HDL___ Total____				LDL___ HDL___ Total____	
		LDL___ HDL___ Total____				LDL___ HDL___ Total____	
		LDL___ HDL___ Total____				LDL___ HDL___ Total____	
		LDL___ HDL___ Total____				LDL___ HDL___ Total____	
		LDL___ HDL___ Total____				LDL___ HDL___ Total____	
		LDL___ HDL___ Total____				LDL___ HDL___ Total____	
		LDL___ HDL___ Total____				LDL___ HDL___ Total____	
		LDL___ HDL___ Total____				LDL___ HDL___ Total____	
		LDL___ HDL___ Total____				LDL___ HDL___ Total____	

DENTAL CARE RECORD

The Dental Care Record is designed to make it easy for you to keep track of every visit to a dentist or dental specialist. For your convenience we've included a section on dental history that should be completed before you visit any dentist for the first time. Use the diagrams of the upper and lower teeth to describe the current status of your teeth. Indicate which teeth are extracted, are filled, have crowns, or are connected with a bridge or partial denture.

In the next section complete the questions concerning particular dental conditions and indicate if they have ever been or are a problem for you. As you review the questions, you are assembling your current dental history or detailing problems you are presently experiencing.

Space is also provided for listing the names and addresses of your current dental practitioners.

Part 3 is your ongoing dental record, to use every time you have an appointment with your dentist. Make sure you describe your symptoms or complaints, using definite terms, such as "third molar on the right side of the lower jaw." Always note if X rays are taken and whether or not they are bite wing (a shot of two or three teeth) or panoramic (a full-mouth shot). List any treatments you have at every visit: for example, a filling, root canal, crown, or gum surgery. Also list the type of filling material used, such as silver amalgam (a mixture of silver and mercury) or acrylic (a plastic type of filling).

If you run out of entry lines, make additional copies of the "Individual Visits" section of this record.

DENTAL CARE RECORD

Complete Part 1 to describe your present state of dental health. Use Part 2 to record the names of your current dental practitioners and Part 3 to record all regularly scheduled and emergency visits to dental practitioners.

Part 1
Dental History

Indicate on the chart below which teeth are decayed, extracted, filled, or crowned. Permanent bridges and partial dentures may be shown by drawing a box around the teeth involved. Use the following symbols: ◨ decayed ⊠ extracted ▬ filled ▢ crown ⊟▭▭▭ bridge or partial denture

UPPER JAW PERMANANT TEETH

LOWER JAW PERMANANT TEETH

Do you have or have you ever had the following?	Treatment/Results
Abscessed tooth	
Bleeding gums	
Broken or bent orthodontic appliance	
Broken or cracked tooth	
Broken or loose crown	
Broken or lost filling	

DENTAL CARE RECORD

Part 1 (Continued)
Dental History

Do you have or have you ever had the following?   **Treatment/Results**

Dentures

Fluoride treatments

Gingivitis (gum inflammation)

Jaw problems
  Broken jaw

  Dislocated jaw

Mouth sores (canker sores)

Occlusion (bite) problems

Root canal

Salivary gland problems

Temporomandibular joint
  (TMJ) problems

Do or did you wear braces?	How long?			
Do or did you wear braces on?	Upper		Lower	Both
Do or did you wear a retainer?	Yes	No	Day	Night

DENTAL CARE RECORD

Part 2
Practitioners

General dentist
Address
Suite
City   St   Zip
Telephone

Orthodontist
Address
Suite
City   St   Zip
Telephone

Endodontist
Address
Suite
City   St   Zip
Telephone

Periodontist
Address
Suite
City   St   Zip
Telephone

Part 3
Individual Dental Visits Record

Date	Practitioner	Symptoms/Complaints/Treatments	X rays taken

Part 3 (Continued)
Individual Dental Visits Record

Date	Practitioner	Symptoms/Complaints/Treatments	X rays taken

Part 3 (Continued)
Individual Dental Visits Record

Date	Practitioner	Symptoms/Complaints/Treatments	X rays taken

Part 3 (Continued)
Individual Dental Visits Record

Date	Practitioner	Symptoms/Complaints/Treatments	X rays taken

DENTAL CARE RECORD

Part 3 (Continued)
Individual Dental Visits Record

Date	Practitioner	Symptoms/Complaints/Treatments	X rays taken

DIAGNOSTIC PROCEDURES RECORD—OUTPATIENT

The Diagnostic Procedures Record—Outpatient is designed for recording the many, varied diagnostic procedures now being performed on an outpatient basis. What this means is that you no longer have to be admitted to the hospital for an overnight stay to have the test or procedure done; doctors' offices, ambulatory facilities, and hospital outpatient departments are common sites. No longer limited to blood tests, outpatient procedures include diagnosis through imaging, such as computed axial tomographic (CAT) scans, magnetic resonance imaging (MRI), nuclear medicine, and ultrasound.

Endoscopic examinations are also commonly performed on an outpatient basis, such as arthroscopy, colonoscopy, and bronchoscopy. (An endoscope is a flexible tube with a light source that enters body orifices or cavities for the purpose of internal examination.)

Enter the date, name and purpose of the procedure, and the name of the practitioner or technician performing it. Depending upon the particular procedure and its purpose, you may have the results right away. Sometimes, however, pieces of tissue are collected and sent for biopsy. In such cases you won't have a complete report by the time you're ready to head home. Enter as much of the results as possible, given what your practitioner has been able to determine.

If there is a follow-up visit, obtain a full report at that time and summarize the results in the appropriate space on the record. As with the Laboratory Tests and Results Record (see page 126), it's a good idea to attach a complete report of the procedure to this record.

DIAGNOSTIC PROCEDURES RECORD—OUTPATIENT

List all diagnostic procedures that you have as an outpatient, including imaging procedures (X ray, CAT scan, MRI, nuclear medicine, and ultrasound), endoscopic examinations, biopsies, EEG, EKG, etc. Enter the date, procedure, setting where performed (ambulatory facility, hospital outpatient department, or doctor's office), purpose and results of the test, and the name of the physician or other practitioner who performed the procedure.

Date	Procedure	Setting where performed	Physician/ Practitioner	Purpose and results

DIAGNOSTIC PROCEDURES RECORD—OUTPATIENT

Date	Procedure	Setting where performed	Physician/ Practitioner	Purpose and results

DIAGNOSTIC PROCEDURES RECORD—OUTPATIENT

Date	Procedure	Setting where performed	Physician/ Practitioner	Purpose and results

DIAGNOSTIC PROCEDURES RECORD—OUTPATIENT

Date	Procedure	Setting where performed	Physician/ Practitioner	Purpose and results

DIAGNOSTIC PROCEDURES RECORD—OUTPATIENT

Date	Procedure	Setting where performed	Physician/ Practitioner	Purpose and results

EMERGENCY DEPARTMENT/ URGICARE CENTER VISITS RECORD

Use this record anytime you receive emergency medical treatment in either the emergency department of a hospital or an urgicare center.

Hospital emergency departments are equipped to handle all life-threatening situations, such as major trauma, cardiac arrest, severed limbs, or severe burns. On the other hand, urgicare centers are designed to provide care for urgent but not life-threatening conditions, such as a sprained ankle, puncture wound, fishhook in finger, severe headache, cough and sore throat, and so on.

This chart enables you to easily record each trip you make to an emergency department or urgicare center. Enter the date and time of your visit and the name of the facility. Summarize the reason for your visit, and record the name of the physician you see and any tests ordered, such as an X ray, blood test, urinalysis, or ultrasound. Enter the results of the tests when reported to you by the practitioner. Because you are in a facility that you may not normally use on a continuing basis, request that copies of all test results be sent to you. Then attach those results to this record.

Once the physician has diagnosed the problem, enter this information on the appropriate lines and summarize any treatment you received. Make note of any special instructions relative to self-care, diet, exercise, bathing, work, or other activities. Also list all medications dispensed at the time of treatment, as well as any prescriptions you received. Remember to also log the name of all medications and prescribed drugs in the Prescription Medications Record (see page 182).

Enter the date and time of any follow-up visit scheduled with either the treating physician or your primary care practitioner.

EMERGENCY DEPARTMENT/URGICARE CENTER
VISITS RECORD

List all visits to hospital emergency departments or urgicare centers, including date and time of visit, name of facility, major complaint or symptoms, name of physician, treatments received, and date of any follow-up visit.

Date   Time   A.M.   P.M.   Facility

Reason for visit

Name of physician

Diagnostic tests ☐ X rays   ☐ Blood test   ☐ Urinalysis   ☐ Ultrasound
Other

Results of tests

Diagnosis and treatment

Special instructions or medications

Date of follow-up visit   Time   A.M.   P.M.

Date   Time   A.M.   P.M.   Facility

Reason for visit

Name of physician

Diagnostic tests ☐ X rays   ☐ Blood test   ☐ Urinalysis   ☐ Ultrasound
Other

Results of tests

Diagnosis and treatment

Special instructions or medications

Date of follow-up visit   Time   A.M.   P.M.

EMERGENCY DEPARTMENT/URGICARE CENTER
VISITS RECORD

Date _____ Time _____ A.M. _____ P.M. _____ Facility _____
Reason for visit _____
Name of physician _____
Diagnostic tests ☐ X rays ☐ Blood test ☐ Urinalysis ☐ Ultrasound
Other _____

Results of tests _____
_____
_____

Diagnosis and treatment _____
_____
_____

Special instructions or medications _____

Date of follow-up visit _____ Time _____ A.M. _____ P.M.

Date _____ Time _____ A.M. _____ P.M. _____ Facility _____
Reason for visit _____
Name of physician _____
Diagnostic tests ☐ X rays ☐ Blood test ☐ Urinalysis ☐ Ultrasound
Other _____

Results of tests _____
_____
_____

Diagnosis and treatment _____
_____
_____

Special instructions or medications _____

Date of follow-up visit _____ Time _____ A.M. _____ P.M.
_____
_____

EMERGENCY DEPARTMENT/URGICARE CENTER VISITS RECORD

Date _____ Time _____ A.M. ___ P.M. ___ Facility _____

Reason for visit _____

Name of physician _____

Diagnostic tests ☐ X rays ☐ Blood test ☐ Urinalysis ☐ Ultrasound

Other _____

Results of tests _____

_____

_____

Diagnosis and treatment _____

_____

_____

Special instructions or medications _____

_____

Date of follow-up visit _____ Time _____ A.M. ___ P.M. ___

Date _____ Time _____ A.M. ___ P.M. ___ Facility _____

Reason for visit _____

Name of physician _____

Diagnostic tests ☐ X rays ☐ Blood test ☐ Urinalysis ☐ Ultrasound

Other _____

Results of tests _____

_____

_____

Diagnosis and treatment _____

_____

_____

Special instructions or medications _____

_____

Date of follow-up visit _____ Time _____ A.M. ___ P.M. ___

EMERGENCY DEPARTMENT/URGICARE CENTER
VISITS RECORD

Date   Time   A.M.   P.M.   Facility

Reason for visit

Name of physician

Diagnostic tests ☐ X rays ☐ Blood test ☐ Urinalysis ☐ Ultrasound

Other

Results of tests

Diagnosis and treatment

Special instructions or medications

Date of follow-up visit   Time   A.M.   P.M.

Date   Time   A.M.   P.M.   Facility

Reason for visit

Name of physician

Diagnostic tests ☐ X rays ☐ Blood test ☐ Urinalysis ☐ Ultrasound

Other

Results of tests

Diagnosis and treatment

Special instructions or medications

Date of follow-up visit   Time   A.M.   P.M.

EMERGENCY DEPARTMENT/URGICARE CENTER
VISITS RECORD

Date _____ Time _____ A.M. ___ P.M. ___ Facility _____

Reason for visit _____

Name of physician _____

Diagnostic tests ☐ X rays ☐ Blood test ☐ Urinalysis ☐ Ultrasound

Other _____

Results of tests _____

_____

Diagnosis and treatment _____

_____

_____

Special instructions or medications _____

_____

Date of follow-up visit _____ Time _____ A.M. ___ P.M. ___

_____

Date _____ Time _____ A.M. ___ P.M. ___ Facility _____

Reason for visit _____

Name of physician _____

Diagnostic tests ☐ X rays ☐ Blood test ☐ Urinalysis ☐ Ultrasound

Other _____

Results of tests _____

_____

Diagnosis and treatment _____

_____

Special instructions or medications _____

_____

Date of follow-up visit _____ Time _____ A.M. ___ P.M. ___

EMERGENCY DEPARTMENT/URGICARE CENTER
VISITS RECORD

Date _____ Time _____ A.M. ___ P.M. ___ Facility _____

Reason for visit _____

Name of physician _____

Diagnostic tests ☐ X rays ☐ Blood test ☐ Urinalysis ☐ Ultrasound

Other _____

Results of tests _____

_____

_____

Diagnosis and treatment _____

_____

_____

Special instructions or medications _____

_____

Date of follow-up visit _____ Time _____ A.M. ___ P.M. ___

_____

Date _____ Time _____ A.M. ___ P.M. ___ Facility _____

Reason for visit _____

Name of physician _____

Diagnostic tests ☐ X rays ☐ Blood test ☐ Urinalysis ☐ Ultrasound

Other _____

Results of tests _____

_____

_____

Diagnosis and treatment _____

_____

_____

Special instructions or medications _____

_____

Date of follow-up visit _____ Time _____ A.M. ___ P.M. ___

_____

EMERGENCY DEPARTMENT/URGICARE CENTER
VISITS RECORD

Date _____ Time _____ A.M. _____ P.M. _____ Facility _____

Reason for visit _____

Name of physician _____

Diagnostic tests ☐ X rays ☐ Blood test ☐ Urinalysis ☐ Ultrasound

Other _____

Results of tests _____

_____

_____

Diagnosis and treatment _____

_____

_____

Special instructions or medications _____

_____

Date of follow-up visit _____ Time _____ A.M. _____ P.M. _____

Date _____ Time _____ A.M. _____ P.M. _____ Facility _____

Reason for visit _____

Name of physician _____

Diagnostic tests ☐ X rays ☐ Blood test ☐ Urinalysis ☐ Ultrasound

Other _____

Results of tests _____

_____

_____

Diagnosis and treatment _____

_____

_____

Special instructions or medications _____

_____

Date of follow-up visit _____ Time _____ A.M. _____ P.M. _____

HOSPITAL RECORD

The Hospital Record enables you to keep track of everything that happens to you during a hospitalization and includes a daily log for you to detail who does what and when.

You will be able to enter some of the information requested in Part 1 at the time of your admission to the hospital—date of admission, name of hospital, and names of your admitting physician and any consulting physician(s) assigned to your case. Obviously, other entries in Part 1—diagnostic tests ordered and your discharge date, for example—must wait until later in your hospitalization.

Part 2, the Daily Hospitalization Record, asks you to keep a daily record of visits to your room by your medical professionals and the vast array of hospital personnel. With this log you will be able to see—and to demonstrate, if need be, at the cashier's office or in the courtroom—whether the anesthesiologist showed up as he recorded, if the administrator really did drop by to chat about your complaints, and how often your doctor poked her nose in the door to see how you were doing. Remember that in a medical setting, as in life, people don't always do what they say they are going to do; or they might even do something and then say they didn't.

Make sure this log is accurate. It may come in very handy somewhere up the road. Enter the date and time of the service or medication you received and the name of the person who provided the service. Another item to note in the daily log is the amount of time it takes for the nurses to respond when you call. As you complete the daily record, you may discover that there's something lacking in the care you are receiving, and you can bring this to the attention of your physician or the hospital administrator.

Keep all entries in chronological order to make it easier to check a particular day of your hospital stay.

HOSPITAL RECORD

In Part 1 list all major hospitalizations, including dates of admission and discharge, admitting physician, consulting physician(s), reason for admission, diagnosis, treatments, and so on. Use a separate page for each period of hospitalization. In Part 2 record the daily activities that accompany your hospitalization. Keep all admissions in chronological order.

Part 1
Personal Data

Date	Admitted	Discharged
Hospital		
Address		
City	St Zip	Telephone
Admitting physician		Telephone
Consulting physician(s)		Telephone
		Telephone
		Telephone
Surgeon(s)		Telephone
		Telephone

Reason for admission

Diagnosis and treatments

Discharged to ☐ Home
          ☐ Nursing home
          ☐ Other facility

HOSPITAL RECORD

Part 2
Daily Hospitalization Record

Use this section to list the services you receive while hospitalized.
Enter the date and time of each service, including physician visits,
diagnostic procedures, medications administered, treatments
undergone, and so on. Be sure to include the name of the person
who provides the service. Also list all time spent in special care
units, such as an intensive care, cardiac care, or burn care unit.

Date	Time	Service or procedure provided	Name of person

HOSPITAL RECORD

Date	Time	Service or procedure provided	Name of person

HOSPITAL RECORD

Date	Time	Service or procedure provided	Name of person

HOSPITAL RECORD

Date	Time	Service or procedure provided	Name of person

HOSPITAL RECORD

In Part 1 list all major hospitalizations, including dates of admission and discharge, admitting physician, consulting physician(s), reason for admission, diagnosis, treatments, and so on. Use a separate page for each period of hospitalization. In Part 2 record the daily activities that accompany your hospitalization. Keep all admissions in chronological order.

Part 1
Personal Data

Date   Admitted   Discharged
Hospital
Address
City   St   Zip   Telephone
Admitting physician   Telephone
Consulting physician(s)   Telephone
                                             Telephone
                                             Telephone
Surgeon(s)   Telephone
                                             Telephone
Reason for admission
_____
_____
_____
_____
_____

Diagnosis and treatments
_____
_____
_____
_____
_____
_____
_____
_____

Discharged to   ☐ Home
        ☐ Nursing home
        ☐ Other facility
_____
_____

HOSPITAL RECORD

Part 2
Daily Hospitalization Record

Use this section to list the services you receive while hospitalized.
Enter the date and time of each service, including physician visits,
diagnostic procedures, medications administered, treatments
undergone, and so on. Be sure to include the name of the person
who provides the service. Also list all time spent in special care
units, such as an intensive care, cardiac care, or burn care unit.

Date	Time	Service or procedure provided	Name of person

HOSPITAL RECORD

Date	Time	Service or procedure provided	Name of person

HOSPITAL RECORD

Date	Time	Service or procedure provided	Name of person

HOSPITAL RECORD

Date	Time	Service or procedure provided	Name of person

HOSPITAL RECORD

In Part 1 list all major hospitalizations, including dates of admission and discharge, admitting physician, consulting physician(s), reason for admission, diagnosis, treatments, and so on. Use a separate page for each period of hospitalization. In Part 2 record the daily activities that accompany your hospitalization. Keep all admissions in chronological order.

Part 1
Personal Data

Date	Admitted	Discharged
Hospital		
Address		
City	St Zip	Telephone
Admitting physician		Telephone
Consulting physician(s)		Telephone
		Telephone
		Telephone
Surgeon(s)		Telephone
		Telephone

Reason for admission

Diagnosis and treatments

Discharged to ☐ Home
　　　☐ Nursing home
　　　☐ Other facility

Part 2
Daily Hospitalization Record

Use this section to list the services you receive while hospitalized.
Enter the date and time of each service, including physician visits,
diagnostic procedures, medications administered, treatments
undergone, and so on. Be sure to include the name of the person
who provides the service. Also list all time spent in special care
units, such as an intensive care, cardiac care, or burn care unit.

Date	Time	Service or procedure provided	Name of person

HOSPITAL RECORD

Date	Time	Service or procedure provided	Name of person

HOSPITAL RECORD

Date	Time	Service or procedure provided	Name of person

HOSPITAL RECORD

Date	Time	Service or procedure provided	Name of person

HOSPITAL RECORD

In Part 1 list all major hospitalizations, including dates of admission and discharge, admitting physician, consulting physician(s), reason for admission, diagnosis, treatments, and so on. Use a separate page for each period of hospitalization. In Part 2 record the daily activities that accompany your hospitalization. Keep all admissions in chronological order.

Part 1
Personal Data

Date	Admitted	Discharged
Hospital		
Address		
City	St Zip	Telephone
Admitting physician		Telephone
Consulting physician(s)		Telephone
		Telephone
		Telephone
Surgeon(s)		Telephone
		Telephone

Reason for admission

Diagnosis and treatments

Discharged to ☐ Home
☐ Nursing home
☐ Other facility

HOSPITAL RECORD

Part 2
Daily Hospitalization Record

Use this section to list the services you receive while hospitalized.
Enter the date and time of each service, including physician visits,
diagnostic procedures, medications administered, treatments
undergone, and so on. Be sure to include the name of the person
who provides the service. Also list all time spent in special care
units, such as an intensive care, cardiac care, or burn care unit.

Date	Time	Service or procedure provided	Name of person

HOSPITAL RECORD

Date	Time	Service or procedure provided	Name of person

HOSPITAL RECORD

Date	Time	Service or procedure provided	Name of person

HOSPITAL RECORD

Date	Time	Service or procedure provided	Name of person

HOSPITAL RECORD

In Part 1 list all major hospitalizations, including dates of admission and discharge, admitting physician, consulting physician(s), reason for admission, diagnosis, treatments, and so on. Use a separate page for each period of hospitalization. In Part 2 record the daily activities that accompany your hospitalization. Keep all admissions in chronological order.

Part 1
Personal Data

Date   Admitted   Discharged

Hospital

Address

City   St   Zip   Telephone

Admitting physician   Telephone

Consulting physician(s)   Telephone

                                                 Telephone

                                                 Telephone

Surgeon(s)   Telephone

                                                 Telephone

Reason for admission

Diagnosis and treatments

Discharged to ☐ Home
          ☐ Nursing home
          ☐ Other facility

HOSPITAL RECORD

Part 2
Daily Hospitalization Record

Use this section to list the services you receive while hospitalized.
Enter the date and time of each service, including physician visits,
diagnostic procedures, medications administered, treatments
undergone, and so on. Be sure to include the name of the person
who provides the service. Also list all time spent in special care
units, such as an intensive care, cardiac care, or burn care unit.

Date	Time	Service or procedure provided	Name of person

HOSPITAL RECORD

Date	Time	Service or procedure provided	Name of person

HOSPITAL RECORD

Date	Time	Service or procedure provided	Name of person

HOSPITAL RECORD

Date	Time	Service or procedure provided	Name of person

HOSPITAL RECORD
(MILITARY AND VETERANS HOSPITALS)

This record may be used by active duty or retired military personnel to summarize the time spent in military and veterans hospitals. Enter the dates of admission and discharge and the reason for your hospitalization. Also include the name of your admitting physician and any consulting physicians involved in your care.

Indicate by check mark the major diagnostic tests or other diagnostic procedures you had. Enter the results of these tests and procedures in the space provided. It is also a good idea to obtain copies of the laboratory reports and attach them to this record.

Maintaining your own military hospital record is a safeguard against having your official record lost when you transfer from one duty station to another. Former military personnel eligible for care at Veterans Administration health facilities should maintain their own records for much the same reason.

Active duty personnel may obtain copies of their medical records from the post hospital under the federal Privacy Act and Freedom of Information Act. Former and retired military personnel may obtain copies of older medical records from the National Archives Record Center, located in St. Louis. See "Accessing Your Medical Records" (page 8) for more information on how to obtain military medical records.

HOSPITAL RECORD
(MILITARY AND VETERANS HOSPITALS)

List your major hospitalizations, including dates of admission and discharge, reason for admission, admitting physician, diagnostic procedures, diagnosis, and treatments. Keep all admissions in chronological order.

Date Admitted _____ Discharged _____

Facility _____

Reason for admission _____

Admitting physician _____

Consulting physician(s) _____

Surgeon(s) _____

Diagnostic tests ☐ X rays ☐ Blood test ☐ Urinalysis ☐ Ultrasound

Other _____

Results _____

Date Admitted _____ Discharged _____

Facility _____

Reason for admission _____

Admitting physician _____

Consulting physician(s) _____

Surgeon(s) _____

Diagnostic tests ☐ X rays ☐ Blood test ☐ Urinalysis ☐ Ultrasound

Other _____

Results _____

HOSPITAL RECORD
(MILITARY AND VETERANS HOSPITALS)

Date Admitted _____ Discharged _____
Facility _____

Reason for admission _____

Admitting physician _____
Consulting physician(s) _____

Surgeon(s) _____

Diagnostic tests ☐ X rays ☐ Blood test ☐ Urinalysis ☐ Ultrasound
Other _____

Results _____

Date Admitted _____ Discharged _____
Facility _____

Reason for admission _____

Admitting physician _____
Consulting physician(s) _____

Surgeon(s) _____

Diagnostic tests ☐ X rays ☐ Blood test ☐ Urinalysis ☐ Ultrasound
Other _____

Results _____

HOSPITAL RECORD
(MILITARY AND VETERANS HOSPITALS)

Date Admitted _____ Discharged _____
Facility _____

Reason for admission _____
_____

Admitting physician _____
Consulting physician(s) _____

Surgeon(s) _____

Diagnostic tests ☐ X rays ☐ Blood test ☐ Urinalysis ☐ Ultrasound
Other _____
_____

Results _____
_____
_____
_____

Date Admitted _____ Discharged _____
Facility _____

Reason for admission _____
_____

Admitting physician _____
Consulting physician(s) _____

Surgeon(s) _____

Diagnostic tests ☐ X rays ☐ Blood test ☐ Urinalysis ☐ Ultrasound
Other _____
_____

Results _____
_____
_____
_____

HOSPITAL RECORD
(MILITARY AND VETERANS HOSPITALS)

Date Admitted   Discharged
Facility

Reason for admission

Admitting physician
Consulting physician(s)

Surgeon(s)

Diagnostic tests ☐ X rays ☐ Blood test ☐ Urinalysis ☐ Ultrasound
Other

Results

Date Admitted   Discharged
Facility

Reason for admission

Admitting physician
Consulting physician(s)

Surgeon(s)

Diagnostic tests ☐ X rays ☐ Blood test ☐ Urinalysis ☐ Ultrasound
Other

Results

HOSPITAL RECORD
(MILITARY AND VETERANS HOSPITALS)

Date Admitted   Discharged

Facility

Reason for admission

Admitting physician

Consulting physician(s)

Surgeon(s)

Diagnostic tests ☐ X rays ☐ Blood test ☐ Urinalysis ☐ Ultrasound

Other

Results

Date Admitted   Discharged

Facility

Reason for admission

Admitting physician

Consulting physician(s)

Surgeon(s)

Diagnostic tests ☐ X rays ☐ Blood test ☐ Urinalysis ☐ Ultrasound

Other

Results

INDIVIDUAL GYNECOLOGICAL RECORD

The Individual Gynecological Record is used each time you visit your practitioner—whether a gynecologist, family doctor, or nurse-midwife—for an examination, for diagnostic tests, and to receive specific treatments.

Use Part 1 to complete your individual gynecological history. If you have already completed the Family Obstetrical and Gynecological History, you should recognize the list of conditions or problems, because they are identical to those listed there. Place a check mark next to those conditions or problems that you experience or have experienced.

Use Part 2 for recording the names, addresses, and telephone numbers of your current gynecological practitioner(s). We suggest that you make all entries in pencil since you may not always have the same practitioner(s).

In Part 3 detail each visit. Enter the date of your appointment, practitioner seen, reason for visit (describe your symptoms or complaints), diagnostic procedures performed or ordered, results of examination, diagnosis and treatment, special instructions, and the date of your next visit. Make sure you keep all visits in chronological order; this enables you to have a more accurate and accessible record of your gynecological health. If you anticipate making several visits to different practitioners, you should make extra copies of Part 3, since this section is used on a continuous basis.

INDIVIDUAL GYNECOLOGICAL RECORD

Part 1
Gynecological Checklist

Indicate by check mark those conditions or problems that you experience and your age at onset.

Condition/Problem	Age	Condition/Problem	Age
Abnormal breast exam		Menopause	
Abnormal Pap smear		Miscarriage	
Abnormal pelvic exam		Painful breasts	
Abortion (elective)		Painful intercourse	
Age began menstruating		Painful menstruation	
Average number of days in cycle		Pregnancies	
Average length of period		Premenstrual symptoms	
Birth control pills		Sexual dissatisfaction	
Bleeding between periods		Sexually transmitted diseases	
Breast biopsy		Tubal ligation	
Cervical biopsy		Tumors—breasts	
Colposcopy		Tumors—ovaries	
DES (diethylstilbestrol) exposure		Tumors—uterus	
Endometrial biopsy		Vaginal infections	
Fragile bones		Other conditions	
Hormone replacement therapy			
IUD			

Part 2
Gynecological Practitioners

Enter the name(s) of your current gynecological practitioner(s).

Gynecologist
Address   Suite
City   St   Zip   Telephone

Nurse-midwife
Address   Suite
City   St   Zip   Telephone

Family/Primary care physician
Address   Suite
City   St   Zip   Telephone

INDIVIDUAL GYNECOLOGICAL RECORD

Part 3
Gynecological Visits Record

Complete the information requested for each visit to your practitioner. Use descriptive terms for your symptoms, such as *pain, irregular bleeding, abdominal swelling,* etc.

Date _____ Practitioner seen _____
Reason for visit (describe your symptoms) _____

Diagnostic procedures _____

Results of examination _____

Diagnosis and treatment _____

Special instructions _____

Date of next scheduled visit _____ Time _____ A.M. _____ P.M.

Date _____ Practitioner seen _____
Reason for visit (describe your symptoms) _____

Diagnostic procedures _____

Results of examination _____

Diagnosis and treatment _____

Special instructions _____

Date of next scheduled visit _____ Time _____ A.M. _____ P.M.

INDIVIDUAL GYNECOLOGICAL RECORD

Part 3 (Continued)
Gynecological Visits Record

Date   Practitioner seen

Reason for visit (describe your symptoms)

Diagnostic procedures

Results of examination

Diagnosis and treatment

Special instructions

Date of next scheduled visit   Time   A.M.   P.M.

Date   Practitioner seen

Reason for visit (describe your symptoms)

Diagnostic procedures

Results of examination

Diagnosis and treatment

Special instructions

Date of next scheduled visit   Time   A.M.   P.M.

Part 3 (Continued)
Gynecological Visits Record

Date   Practitioner seen
Reason for visit (describe your symptoms)

Diagnostic procedures

Results of examination

Diagnosis and treatment

Special instructions

Date of next scheduled visit   Time   A.M.   P.M.

Date   Practitioner seen
Reason for visit (describe your symptoms)

Diagnostic procedures

Results of examination

Diagnosis and treatment

Special instructions

Date of next scheduled visit   Time   A.M.   P.M.

Part 3 (Continued)
Gynecological Visits Record

Date _____ Practitioner seen _____

Reason for visit (describe your symptoms) _____

Diagnostic procedures _____

Results of examination _____

Diagnosis and treatment _____

Special instructions _____

Date of next scheduled visit _____ Time _____ A.M. _____ P.M. _____

Date _____ Practitioner seen _____

Reason for visit (describe your symptoms) _____

Diagnostic procedures _____

Results of examination _____

Diagnosis and treatment _____

Special instructions _____

Date of next scheduled visit _____ Time _____ A.M. _____ P.M. _____

Part 3 (Continued)
Gynecological Visits Record

Date _____ Practitioner seen _____

Reason for visit (describe your symptoms) _____

_____

Diagnostic procedures _____

Results of examination _____

_____

Diagnosis and treatment _____

_____

Special instructions _____

_____

Date of next scheduled visit _____ Time _____ A.M. _____ P.M. _____

Date _____ Practitioner seen _____

Reason for visit (describe your symptoms) _____

_____

Diagnostic procedures _____

Results of examination _____

_____

Diagnosis and treatment _____

_____

Special instructions _____

_____

Date of next scheduled visit _____ Time _____ A.M. _____ P.M. _____

Part 3 (Continued)
Gynecological Visits Record

Date   Practitioner seen

Reason for visit (describe your symptoms)

Diagnostic procedures

Results of examination

Diagnosis and treatment

Special instructions

Date of next scheduled visit   Time   A.M.   P.M.

Date   Practitioner seen

Reason for visit (describe your symptoms)

Diagnostic procedures

Results of examination

Diagnosis and treatment

Special instructions

Date of next scheduled visit   Time   A.M.   P.M.

Part 3 (Continued)
Gynecological Visits Record

Date   Practitioner seen
Reason for visit (describe your symptoms)

Diagnostic procedures

Results of examination

Diagnosis and treatment

Special instructions

Date of next scheduled visit   Time   A.M.   P.M.

Date   Practitioner seen
Reason for visit (describe your symptoms)

Diagnostic procedures

Results of examination

Diagnosis and treatment

Special instructions

Date of next scheduled visit   Time   A.M.   P.M.

INDIVIDUAL GYNECOLOGICAL RECORD

Part 3 (Continued)
Gynecological Visits Record

Date _____ Practitioner seen _____
Reason for visit (describe your symptoms) _____

Diagnostic procedures _____

Results of examination _____

Diagnosis and treatment _____

Special instructions _____

Date of next scheduled visit _____ Time _____ A.M. _____ P.M.

Date _____ Practitioner seen _____
Reason for visit (describe your symptoms) _____

Diagnostic procedures _____

Results of examination _____

Diagnosis and treatment _____

Special instructions _____

Date of next scheduled visit _____ Time _____ A.M. _____ P.M.

INDIVIDUAL GYNECOLOGICAL RECORD

Part 3 (Continued)
Gynecological Visits Record

Date   Practitioner seen
Reason for visit (describe your symptoms)

Diagnostic procedures

Results of examination

Diagnosis and treatment

Special instructions

Date of next scheduled visit   Time   A.M.   P.M.

Date   Practitioner seen
Reason for visit (describe your symptoms)

Diagnostic procedures

Results of examination

Diagnosis and treatment

Special instructions

Date of next scheduled visit   Time   A.M.   P.M.

INDIVIDUAL GYNECOLOGICAL RECORD

Part 3 (Continued)
Gynecological Visits Record

Date   Practitioner seen
Reason for visit (describe your symptoms)

Diagnostic procedures

Results of examination

Diagnosis and treatment

Special instructions

Date of next scheduled visit   Time   A.M.   P.M.

Date   Practitioner seen
Reason for visit (describe your symptoms)

Diagnostic procedures

Results of examination

Diagnosis and treatment

Special instructions

Date of next scheduled visit   Time   A.M.   P.M.

INDIVIDUAL PRACTITIONER VISITS RECORD

The Individual Practitioner Visits Record is integral to your complete medical record; indeed, it's the one you'll probably use more than any other. It allows you to record each and every detail of every visit to just about any medical practitioner you see—your primary care physician, as well as specialists. Use it, too, for visits to a podiatrist, chiropractor, psychologist or counselor, nutritionist, and so on. You would not use this form, however, for dental, obstetrical/gynecological, or vision care visits since there are special records for those practitioners.

Begin your record by entering the date of your visit and the name of your practitioner. Next, enter your symptoms and complaints. Try to be as descriptive and accurate as possible when you do this. Don't just say "pain," for example, but be more specific. Descriptive phrases, such as "sharp pain on the right side of the lower abdomen" or "chest pain in the upper left near the shoulder," help your practitioner narrow the field of possibilities. Also enter any temperature, pulse, or blood pressure measurements taken if relevant to your symptoms or complaints.

When your practitioner examines you, note what he or she is doing. Ask for specific reports regarding your blood pressure, temperature, pulse, respiration, or chest sounds. If you're given an order for laboratory tests or a diagnostic procedure, enter that information here, in the Laboratory Tests and Results Record (see page 126), and in the Diagnostic Procedures Record—Outpatient (see page 54).

Make sure your practitioner gives you a diagnosis and record it in the column "Diagnosis and Treatment." Also enter any treatment received, including injections, spinal manipulations or adjustments, foreign objects removed, growths excised, and so on. Remember, too, that medication is a form of treatment, so record all medications dispensed and prescriptions received at this visit. Also enter the information in the Prescription Medications Record (see page 182) after you have the prescription filled at your pharmacy.

INDIVIDUAL PRACTITIONER VISITS RECORD

List all visits to any medical practitioner, including your primary care physician, any specialists, chiropractor, podiatrist, nutritionist, and so on. Enter the date, practitioner's name and address, symptoms/complaints, and diagnosis and treatment.

Date	Practitioner Name and Address	Symptoms/Complaints	Diagnosis and treatment

INDIVIDUAL PRACTITIONER VISITS RECORD

Date	Practitioner Name and Address	Symptoms/Complaints	Diagnosis and treatment

INDIVIDUAL PRACTITIONER VISITS RECORD

Date	Practitioner Name and Address	Symptoms/Complaints	Diagnosis and treatment

INDIVIDUAL PRACTITIONER VISITS RECORD

Date	Practitioner Name and Address	Symptoms/Complaints	Diagnosis and treatment

INDIVIDUAL PRACTITIONER VISITS RECORD

Date	Practitioner Name and Address	Symptoms/Complaints	Diagnosis and treatment

INDIVIDUAL PRACTITIONER VISITS RECORD

Date	Practitioner Name and Address	Symptoms/Complaints	Diagnosis and treatment

INDIVIDUAL PRACTITIONER VISITS RECORD

Date	Practitioner Name and Address	Symptoms/Complaints	Diagnosis and treatment

INDIVIDUAL PRACTITIONER VISITS RECORD

Date	Practitioner Name and Address	Symptoms/Complaints	Diagnosis and treatment

INDIVIDUAL PRACTITIONER VISITS RECORD

Date	Practitioner Name and Address	Symptoms/Complaints	Diagnosis and treatment

INDIVIDUAL PRACTITIONER VISITS RECORD

Date	Practitioner Name and Address	Symptoms/Complaints	Diagnosis and treatment

INDIVIDUAL PRACTITIONER VISITS RECORD

Date	Practitioner Name and Address	Symptoms/Complaints	Diagnosis and treatment

INDIVIDUAL PRACTITIONER VISITS RECORD

Date	Practitioner Name and Address	Symptoms/Complaints	Diagnosis and treatment

INDIVIDUAL PRACTITIONER VISITS RECORD

Date	Practitioner Name and Address	Symptoms/Complaints	Diagnosis and treatment

LABORATORY TESTS AND RESULTS RECORD

Use the Laboratory Tests and Results Record to track all diagnostic tests ordered by your practitioner. Enter the date and name of the test, laboratory performing the test, practitioner who ordered the test, and, if appropriate, the name of the person performing it. If you're unfamiliar with the name of the test, ask your practitioner for clarification. Unless this is a test that shows immediate results, you won't know the outcome until your next scheduled visit to your practitioner.

At this next visit, make sure you get a copy of the report, even if your practitioner has already gone over the results with you. Then summarize the results of the test in the appropriate column and attach the report to this record. The more information you have at your fingertips, the better informed and educated a medical consumer you will become.

LABORATORY TESTS AND RESULTS RECORD

List all lab tests that you have, including the date, name of the test, laboratory performing the test, results of the test, and the name of the physician who ordered the test. Attach a copy of the lab results to this record.

Date	Test ordered	Laboratory	Results	Physician

LABORATORY TESTS AND RESULTS RECORD

Date	Test ordered	Laboratory	Results	Physician

LABORATORY TESTS AND RESULTS RECORD

Date	Test ordered	Laboratory	Results	Physician

LABORATORY TESTS AND RESULTS RECORD

Date	Test ordered	Laboratory	Results	Physician

LABORATORY TESTS AND RESULTS RECORD

Date	Test ordered	Laboratory	Results	Physician

LABORATORY TESTS AND RESULTS RECORD

Date	Test ordered	Laboratory	Results	Physician

LABORATORY TESTS AND RESULTS RECORD

Date	Test ordered	Laboratory	Results	Physician

NURSING HOME RECORD

The Nursing Home Record makes it easy for you to keep an accurate summary of your stay—or the stay of someone for whom you are acting as advocate—in a nursing home. The term nursing home is actually a very general name for several different types of medical care facilities. It has the connotation of being a "last stop" for the elderly, but it actually can be a place for people of all ages to convalesce following an accident or serious illness, or a temporary placement for an elderly person while the family shops around and lines up alternative modes of care.

Whatever your particular need, begin by entering the dates of your admission and discharge, name of the facility, address, city, state, zip, and telephone. (If you're unable to complete this, ask a family member or other relative or friend to assist you.) Next, enter the level of care you received during your stay, whether skilled, intermediate, or custodial. Skilled care is delivered by registered and licensed practical nurses on the orders of an attending physician (most likely your personal physician). This is the most intensive level of care available, and usually indicates that you are bedridden and require constant nursing services, such as intravenous medications, change of surgical dressing, or inhalation therapy. Skilled care may be for a short or extended period of time.

Less intensive than skilled care, intermediate care is for those people who are not bedridden but have some degree of mobility. Here, too, care is delivered by registered and licensed practical nurses and an array of therapists. This care stresses rehabilitation therapy to enable a person to regain a certain functional level and return to his or her home.

Custodial care is nonmedical, which means you do not require constant attention from nurses or other medical personnel but do require assistance with activities of daily living, such as getting out of bed, walking, eating, and bathing. Custodial care is usually provided on a long-term basis.

In this section indicate by check mark the level that comes closest to the care you received.

Indicate the method of payment for your stay: nursing home

insurance, Medicaid, Medicare, or private payment. Remember, some forms of nursing home coverage are limited, such as Medicare, which covers only skilled care and only for a limited number of days. Therefore, it's possible that you began your stay under one coverage and at some point switched to a different coverage at the time of discharge.

Enter the names and telephone numbers of the admitting physician, facility medical director, and facility administrator. You want these important telephone numbers available in the event there's a problem with the care you receive.

Finally, summarize the reason you required this particular nursing home stay. Also note whether you were discharged to your home, hospital, or another facility.

NURSING HOME RECORD

List all periods of time spent in nursing homes, including dates of admission and discharge, level of care received, and admitting physician.

Date Admitted   Discharged

Facility

Address

City   St   Zip

Telephone

Level of care received   ☐ Skilled   ☐ Intermediate   ☐ Custodial

Method of payment

    ☐ Private insurance ☐ Medicaid ☐ Medicare ☐ Private payment

Admitting physician   Telephone

Facility medical director   Telephone

Facility administrator   Telephone

Reason for admission

Discharged to ☐ Home

    ☐ Hospital

    ☐ Other facility

Date Admitted   Discharged

Facility

Address

City   St   Zip

Telephone

Level of care received   ☐ Skilled   ☐ Intermediate   ☐ Custodial

Method of payment

    ☐ Private insurance ☐ Medicaid ☐ Medicare ☐ Private payment

Admitting physician   Telephone

Facility medical director   Telephone

Facility administrator   Telephone

Reason for admission

Discharged to ☐ Home

    ☐ Hospital

    ☐ Other facility

NURSING HOME RECORD

Date Admitted _____ Discharged _____
Facility _____
Address _____

City _____ St _____ Zip _____
Telephone _____
Level of care received ☐ Skilled ☐ Intermediate ☐ Custodial
Method of payment
☐ Private insurance ☐ Medicaid ☐ Medicare ☐ Private payment
Admitting physician _____ Telephone _____
Facility medical director _____ Telephone _____
Facility administrator _____ Telephone _____
Reason for admission _____

Discharged to ☐ Home
☐ Hospital
☐ Other facility

Date Admitted _____ Discharged _____
Facility _____
Address _____

City _____ St _____ Zip _____
Telephone _____
Level of care received ☐ Skilled ☐ Intermediate ☐ Custodial
Method of payment
☐ Private insurance ☐ Medicaid ☐ Medicare ☐ Private payment
Admitting physician _____ Telephone _____
Facility medical director _____ Telephone _____
Facility administrator _____ Telephone _____
Reason for admission _____

Discharged to ☐ Home
☐ Hospital
☐ Other facility

NURSING HOME RECORD

Date Admitted _____ Discharged _____

Facility _____

Address _____

City _____ St ___ Zip ___

Telephone _____

Level of care received ☐ Skilled ☐ Intermediate ☐ Custodial

Method of payment

☐ Private insurance ☐ Medicaid ☐ Medicare ☐ Private payment

Admitting physician _____ Telephone _____

Facility medical director _____ Telephone _____

Facility administrator _____ Telephone _____

Reason for admission _____

Discharged to ☐ Home

☐ Hospital

☐ Other facility

Date Admitted _____ Discharged _____

Facility _____

Address _____

City _____ St ___ Zip ___

Telephone _____

Level of care received ☐ Skilled ☐ Intermediate ☐ Custodial

Method of payment

☐ Private insurance ☐ Medicaid ☐ Medicare ☐ Private payment

Admitting physician _____ Telephone _____

Facility medical director _____ Telephone _____

Facility administrator _____ Telephone _____

Reason for admission _____

Discharged to ☐ Home

☐ Hospital

☐ Other facility

NURSING HOME RECORD

Date Admitted   Discharged

Facility

Address

City   St   Zip

Telephone

Level of care received ☐ Skilled   ☐ Intermediate   ☐ Custodial

Method of payment

    ☐ Private insurance ☐ Medicaid ☐ Medicare ☐ Private payment

Admitting physician   Telephone

Facility medical director   Telephone

Facility administrator   Telephone

Reason for admission

Discharged to ☐ Home
    ☐ Hospital
    ☐ Other facility

Date Admitted   Discharged

Facility

Address

City   St   Zip

Telephone

Level of care received ☐ Skilled   ☐ Intermediate   ☐ Custodial

Method of payment

    ☐ Private insurance ☐ Medicaid ☐ Medicare ☐ Private payment

Admitting physician   Telephone

Facility medical director   Telephone

Facility administrator   Telephone

Reason for admission

Discharged to ☐ Home
    ☐ Hospital
    ☐ Other facility

OVER-THE-COUNTER (OTC) MEDICATIONS RECORD

Over-the-counter, or nonprescription, medications play a large role in self-care. OTCs, however, aren't sugar pills; they're real medicines and, as such, can cause real problems if not properly used and monitored. Some of today's popular OTCs were once prescription medications (Afrin nasal spray and Actifed, an antihistamine/decongestant, just to name two examples), and the major pharmaceutical manufacturers are continually pushing the Food and Drug Administration to speed the approval of even more products for the over-the-counter market. So treat these medications as you would those parceled out by your doctor and pharmacist—with caution and a wary eye to safety.

Enter the date you purchased the product in the first column on the form. Next, enter the name of the product, such as Bayer aspirin or Vick's cough syrup.

The expiration date is very important. You don't want to take medications that have gone beyond their expiration dates. Medications begin to deteriorate almost from the moment of manufacture; while not necessarily dangerous, this deterioration can affect the efficacy of the ingredients. So it's best to discard any OTC medications that have gone beyond their expiration dates.

Monitoring the side effects or adverse reactions you experience is a part of learning to be a fully informed medical consumer. Always record any side effects (unwanted effects of the medication, such as dizziness, headache, or dry mouth) or adverse reactions (harmful, potentially life-threatening effects of the medication, such as anaphylactic shock, cardiac arrhythmia, or irregular breathing). When these occur, contact your practitioner or pharmacist immediately. Remember, too, when you purchase over-the-counter drugs to ask the pharmacist about side effects and adverse reactions associated with the products. And be sure to read any warnings on the package.

OVER-THE-COUNTER (OTC) MEDICATIONS RECORD

List all of the OTC medications you purchase, including date purchased, name of medication or product, expiration date, and any side effects (unwanted effects of the medication, such as dizziness, headache, or dry mouth) or adverse reactions (harmful, potentially life-threating effects of the medication, such as anaphylactic shock, cardiac arrhythmia, or irregular breathing) you experience.

Date purchased	Medication/Product	Expiration date	Side effects/Adverse reactions

OVER-THE-COUNTER (OTC) MEDICATIONS RECORD

Date purchased	Medication/Product	Expiration date	Side effects/Adverse reactions

OVER-THE-COUNTER (OTC) MEDICATIONS RECORD

Date purchased	Medication/Product	Expiration date	Side effects/Adverse reactions

OVER-THE-COUNTER (OTC) MEDICATIONS RECORD

Date purchased	Medication/Product	Expiration date	Side effects/Adverse reactions

OVER-THE-COUNTER (OTC) MEDICATIONS RECORD

Date purchased	Medication/Product	Expiration date	Side effects/Adverse reactions

OVER-THE-COUNTER (OTC) MEDICATIONS RECORD

Date purchased	Medication/Product	Expiration date	Side effects/Adverse reactions

Date purchased	Medication/Product	Expiration date	Side effects/Adverse reactions

PRENATAL VISITS RECORD

Use the Prenatal Visits Record to keep track of all pertinent information concerning your pregnancy. As important as it is to be prepared for every medical visit, it's especially critical when you're pregnant and undergoing the many changes that affect both your and your baby's health. So have your research and reading done and your concerns and questions ready.

Why not use this record as Danish women do? They carry their own prenatal records, called "wandering journals," with them to their visits with care-givers. In Part 1 enter the name of your obstetrician, nurse-midwife, or other practitioner. Also enter the name of the facility where you plan to deliver, your age, due date, and the name of someone to notify in case of an emergency.

Part 2 is the nine-month record of your pregnancy. Always enter the date and time of your appointment. Next, enter any symptoms you experience or any questions you wish to ask your practitioner. Record such items as blood pressure and weight measurements, diagnostic procedures performed, or special instructions received. Beginning with your second visit, note the changes that occur from one month to the next in your blood pressure, weight, or anything else that affects your general health (water retention, nausea, or vomiting).

Following the initial (and generally the lengthiest) office visit and calculation of the estimated delivery date, appointments typically are booked as follows:

- From the first visit to 28 weeks, every three to four weeks

- From 28 to 32 weeks, every three weeks

- From 32 to 36 weeks, every two weeks

- From 36 weeks to delivery, once a week

Your schedule may vary somewhat depending upon your general state of health or whether you are considered a high- or low-risk pregnancy.

Part 3 summarizes the birth. Enter the child's name, date of delivery, time of birth, sex, weight, and length. Also record the baby's APGAR score (a test that evaluates the general health of the newborn by examining the heart rate, respiratory effort, muscle tone, response to a tube in the nostril, and color). The normal range for this test is a score of 7 to 9. Also enter your baby's blood type (A, B, AB, or O), including the Rh factor (negative or positive).

Next, enter the place of birth (city and state), facility or setting (hospital, birthing center, or other), and the type of birth (whether vaginal or C-section, full term or premature). Make note of any birthmark, birth defect, or other complication observed at birth. Finally, list the name of the practitioner who assisted with the delivery.

PRENATAL VISITS RECORD

Enter the personal data requested in Part 1, including the name(s) of your birth attendant, facility where you plan to deliver, your age, and due date. Use Part 2 to record your individual visits to your practitioner, and Part 3 to record vital birth information.

Part 1
Personal Data

Name of physician

Address   Suite

City   St   Zip

Telephone

Name of physician

Address   Suite

City   St   Zip

Telephone

Name of Nurse-midwife

Address   Suite

City   St   Zip

Telephone

Facility

Address   Suite

City   St   Zip

Telephone

Is this your first pregnancy? Yes   No   Your age   Due date

In case of emergency, notify

Telephone (home)   (work)

PRENATAL VISITS RECORD

Part 2
Prenatal Visits

Record your weight and blood pressure at each visit and enter any changes from the previous visit. Also list all symptoms you experience and any questions you wish to ask your practitioner at this visit.

Monthly Visits 1st Month	Symptoms/Questions
Date	
Time A.M. P.M.	

Weight   Blood pressure

Diagnostic procedures

Special instructions

Monthly Visits 2nd Month	Symptoms/Questions
Date	
Time A.M. P.M.	

Weight   Blood pressure

Changes from previous visit

Weight   Blood pressure

Diagnostic procedures

Special instructions

Part 2 (Continued)
Prenatal Visits

Monthly Visits 3rd Month	Symptoms/Questions
Date	
Time A.M. P.M.	

Weight	Blood pressure
Changes from previous visit	
Weight	Blood pressure
Diagnostic procedures	

Special instructions

Monthly Visits 4th Month	Symptoms/Questions
Date	
Time A.M. P.M.	

Weight	Blood pressure
Changes from previous visit	
Weight	Blood pressure
Diagnostic procedures	

Special instructions

Part 2 (Continued)
Prenatal Visits

Monthly Visits 5th Month	Symptoms/Questions
Date	
Time A.M. P.M.	

Weight	Blood pressure
Changes from previous visit	
Weight	Blood pressure
Diagnostic procedures	

Special instructions

Monthly Visits 6th Month	Symptoms/Questions
Date	
Time A.M. P.M.	

Weight	Blood pressure
Changes from previous visit	
Weight	Blood pressure
Diagnostic procedures	

Special instructions

Part 2 (Continued)
Prenatal Visits

Monthly Visits 7th Month	Symptoms/Questions
Date	
Time A.M. P.M.	

Weight	Blood pressure
Changes from previous visit	
Weight	Blood pressure
Diagnostic procedures	

Special instructions

Monthly Visits 8th Month	Symptoms/Questions
Date	
Time A.M. P.M.	

Weight	Blood pressure
Changes from previous visit	
Weight	Blood pressure
Diagnostic procedures	

Special instructions

PRENATAL VISITS RECORD

Part 2 (Continued)
Prenatal Visits

Monthly Visits 9th Month	Symptoms/Questions
Date	
Time A.M. P.M.	

Weight	Blood pressure

Changes from previous visit

Weight	Blood pressure

Diagnostic procedures

Special instructions

Other Visits	Symptoms/Questions
Date	
Time A.M. P.M.	

Weight	Blood pressure

Changes from previous visit

Weight	Blood pressure

Diagnostic procedures

Special instructions

Part 2 (Continued)
Prenatal Visits

Other Visits	Symptoms/Questions
Date	
Time A.M. P.M.	

	Weight	Blood pressure
Changes from previous visit		
	Weight	Blood pressure
Diagnostic procedures		

Special instructions

Other Visits	Symptoms/Questions
Date	
Time A.M. P.M.	

	Weight	Blood pressure
Changes from previous visit		
	Weight	Blood pressure
Diagnostic procedures		

Special instructions

Part 3
Birth Summary

Name of child

Date of birth _____ Time of birth _____ A.M. _____ P.M.

Sex ☐ Female ☐ Male

Weight _____ lbs _____ ozs Length _____ inches

APGAR score _____ PKU test _____ Blood type

Place of birth City _____ St

Facility/setting

Hospital

Address

Birthing center

Address

Other

Vaginal birth ☐ Yes ☐ No

C-section ☐ Yes ☐ No

Full term ☐ Yes ☐ No

If no, how many weeks premature

List any birthmark, birth defect, or complication noted at birth

Attending physician

Nurse-midwife

Other practitioner

Other Information

PRENATAL VISITS RECORD

Enter the personal data requested in Part 1, including the name(s) of your birth attendant, facility where you plan to deliver, your age, and due date. Use Part 2 to record your individual visits to your practitioner, and Part 3 to record vital birth information.

Part 1
Personal Data

Name of physician
Address   Suite
City   St   Zip
Telephone

Name of physician
Address   Suite
City   St   Zip
Telephone

Name of Nurse-midwife
Address   Suite
City   St   Zip
Telephone

Facility
Address   Suite
City   St   Zip
Telephone

Is this your first pregnancy? Yes   No   Your age   Due date

In case of emergency, notify

Telephone (home)   (work)

Part 2
Prenatal Visits

Record your weight and blood pressure at each visit and enter any changes from the previous visit. Also list all symptoms you experience and any questions you wish to ask your practitioner at this visit.

Monthly Visits 1st Month	Symptoms/Questions
Date	
Time A.M. P.M.	

Weight   Blood pressure

Diagnostic procedures

Special instructions

Monthly Visits 2nd Month	Symptoms/Questions
Date	
Time A.M. P.M.	

Weight   Blood pressure
Changes from previous visit
Weight   Blood pressure
Diagnostic procedures

Special instructions

Part 2 (Continued)
Prenatal Visits

Monthly Visits 3rd Month	Symptoms/Questions
Date	
Time A.M. P.M.	

Weight	Blood pressure

Changes from previous visit

Weight	Blood pressure

Diagnostic procedures

Special instructions

Monthly Visits 4th Month	Symptoms/Questions
Date	
Time A.M. P.M.	

Weight	Blood pressure

Changes from previous visit

Weight	Blood pressure

Diagnostic procedures

Special instructions

Part 2 (Continued)
Prenatal Visits

Monthly Visits 5th Month	Symptoms/Questions
Date	
Time A.M. P.M.	

Weight	Blood pressure
Changes from previous visit	
Weight	Blood pressure
Diagnostic procedures	

Special instructions

Monthly Visits 6th Month	Symptoms/Questions
Date	
Time A.M. P.M.	

Weight	Blood pressure
Changes from previous visit	
Weight	Blood pressure
Diagnostic procedures	

Special instructions

Part 2 (Continued)
Prenatal Visits

Monthly Visits 7th Month	Symptoms/Questions
Date	
Time A.M. P.M.	

Weight	Blood pressure
Changes from previous visit	
Weight	Blood pressure
Diagnostic procedures	

Special instructions

Monthly Visits 8th Month	Symptoms/Questions
Date	
Time A.M. P.M.	

Weight	Blood pressure
Changes from previous visit	
Weight	Blood pressure
Diagnostic procedures	

Special instructions

Part 2 (Continued)
Prenatal Visits

Monthly Visits 9th Month	Symptoms/Questions
Date	
Time A.M. P.M.	
Weight	Blood pressure
Changes from previous visit	
Weight	Blood pressure
Diagnostic procedures	
Special instructions	

Other Visits	Symptoms/Questions
Date	
Time A.M. P.M.	
Weight	Blood pressure
Changes from previous visit	
Weight	Blood pressure
Diagnostic procedures	
Special instructions	

PRENATAL VISITS RECORD

Part 2 (Continued)
Prenatal Visits

Other Visits	Symptoms/Questions
Date	
Time A.M. P.M.	

Weight   Blood pressure
Changes from previous visit
Weight   Blood pressure
Diagnostic procedures

Special instructions

Other Visits	Symptoms/Questions
Date	
Time A.M. P.M.	

Weight   Blood pressure
Changes from previous visit
Weight   Blood pressure
Diagnostic procedures

Special instructions

PRENATAL VISITS RECORD

Part 3
Birth Summary

Name of child

Date of birth _____ Time of birth _____ A.M. _____ P.M.

Sex ☐ Female ☐ Male

Weight _____ lbs _____ ozs Length _____ inches

APGAR score _____ PKU test _____ Blood type _____

Place of birth City _____ St _____

Facility/setting

Hospital

Address

Birthing center

Address

Other

Vaginal birth ☐ Yes ☐ No

C-section ☐ Yes ☐ No

Full term ☐ Yes ☐ No

If no, how many weeks premature

List any birthmark, birth defect, or complication noted at birth

Attending physician

Nurse-midwife

Other practitioner

Other information

PRENATAL VISITS RECORD

Enter the personal data requested in Part 1, including the name(s) of your birth attendant, facility where you plan to deliver, your age, and due date. Use Part 2 to record your individual visits to your practitioner, and Part 3 to record vital birth information.

Part 1
Personal Data

Name of physician
Address   Suite
City   St   Zip
Telephone

Name of physician
Address   Suite
City   St   Zip
Telephone

Name of Nurse-midwife
Address   Suite
City   St   Zip
Telephone

Facility
Address   Suite
City   St   Zip
Telephone

Is this your first pregnancy? Yes   No   Your age   Due date

In case of emergency, notify

Telephone (home)   (work)

Part 2
Prenatal Visits

Record your weight and blood pressure at each visit and enter any changes from the previous visit. Also list all symptoms you experience and any questions you wish to ask your practitioner at this visit.

Monthly Visits 1st Month	Symptoms/Questions
Date	
Time A.M. P.M.	
Weight Blood pressure	
Diagnostic procedures	
Special instructions	

Monthly Visits 2nd Month	Symptoms/Questions
Date	
Time A.M. P.M.	
Weight Blood pressure	
Changes from previous visit	
Weight Blood pressure	
Diagnostic procedures	
Special instructions	

PRENATAL VISITS RECORD

Part 2 (Continued)
Prenatal Visits

Monthly Visits 3rd Month	Symptoms/Questions
Date	
Time A.M. P.M.	

Weight	Blood pressure
Changes from previous visit	
Weight	Blood pressure
Diagnostic procedures	

Special instructions

Monthly Visits 4th Month	Symptoms/Questions
Date	
Time A.M. P.M.	

Weight	Blood pressure
Changes from previous visit	
Weight	Blood pressure
Diagnostic procedures	

Special instructions

PRENATAL VISITS RECORD

Part 2 (Continued)
Prenatal Visits

Monthly Visits 5th Month	Symptoms/Questions
Date	
Time A.M. P.M.	

Weight	Blood pressure
Changes from previous visit	
Weight	Blood pressure
Diagnostic procedures	

Special instructions

Monthly Visits 6th Month	Symptoms/Questions
Date	
Time A.M. P.M.	

Weight	Blood pressure
Changes from previous visit	
Weight	Blood pressure
Diagnostic procedures	

Special instructions

Part 2 (Continued)
Prenatal Visits

Monthly Visits 7th Month	Symptoms/Questions
Date	
Time A.M. P.M.	

Weight	Blood pressure
Changes from previous visit	
Weight	Blood pressure
Diagnostic procedures	

Special instructions

Monthly Visits 8th Month	Symptoms/Questions
Date	
Time A.M. P.M.	

Weight	Blood pressure
Changes from previous visit	
Weight	Blood pressure
Diagnostic procedures	

Special instructions

Part 2 (Continued)
Prenatal Visits

Monthly Visits 9th Month	Symptoms/Questions
Date	
Time A.M. P.M.	

Weight	Blood pressure
Changes from previous visit	
Weight	Blood pressure
Diagnostic procedures	

Special instructions

___

Other Visits	Symptoms/Questions
Date	
Time A.M. P.M.	

Weight	Blood pressure
Changes from previous visit	
Weight	Blood pressure
Diagnostic procedures	

Special instructions

Part 2 (Continued)
Prenatal Visits

Other Visits	Symptoms/Questions
Date	
Time A.M. P.M.	

Weight   Blood pressure
Changes from previous visit
Weight   Blood pressure
Diagnostic procedures

Special instructions

Other Visits	Symptoms/Questions
Date	
Time A.M. P.M.	

Weight   Blood pressure
Changes from previous visit
Weight   Blood pressure
Diagnostic procedures

Special instructions

PRENATAL VISITS RECORD

Part 3
Birth Summary

Name of child

Date of birth _____ Time of birth _____ A.M. _____ P.M.

Sex ☐ Female ☐ Male

Weight _____ lbs _____ ozs _____ Length _____ inches

APGAR score _____ PKU test _____ Blood type

Place of birth City _____ St

Facility/setting

Hospital

Address

Birthing center

Address

Other

Vaginal birth ☐ Yes ☐ No

C-section ☐ Yes ☐ No

Full term ☐ Yes ☐ No

If no, how many weeks premature

List any birthmark, birth defect, or complication noted at birth

Attending physician

Nurse-midwife

Other practitioner

Other information

PRENATAL VISITS RECORD

Enter the personal data requested in Part 1, including the name(s) of your birth attendant, facility where you plan to deliver, your age, and due date. Use Part 2 to record your individual visits to your practitioner, and Part 3 to record vital birth information.

Part 1
Personal Data

Name of physician

Address   Suite

City   St   Zip

Telephone

Name of physician

Address   Suite

City   St   Zip

Telephone

Name of Nurse-midwife

Address   Suite

City   St   Zip

Telephone

Facility

Address   Suite

City   St   Zip

Telephone

Is this your first pregnancy? Yes   No   Your age   Due date

In case of emergency, notify

Telephone (home)   (work)

PRENATAL VISITS RECORD

Part 2
Prenatal Visits

Record your weight and blood pressure at each visit and enter any changes from the previous visit. Also list all symptoms you experience and any questions you wish to ask your practitioner at this visit.

Monthly Visits 1st Month	Symptoms/Questions
Date	
Time A.M. P.M.	

Weight   Blood pressure

Diagnostic procedures

Special instructions

Monthly Visits 2nd Month	Symptoms/Questions
Date	
Time A.M. P.M.	

Weight   Blood pressure

Changes from previous visit

Weight   Blood pressure

Diagnostic procedures

Special instructions

PRENATAL VISITS RECORD

Part 2 (Continued)
Prenatal Visits

Monthly Visits 3rd Month	Symptoms/Questions
Date	
Time A.M. P.M.	
Weight	Blood pressure
Changes from previous visit	
Weight	Blood pressure
Diagnostic procedures	
Special instructions	

Monthly Visits 4th Month	Symptoms/Questions
Date	
Time A.M. P.M.	
Weight	Blood pressure
Changes from previous visit	
Weight	Blood pressure
Diagnostic procedures	
Special instructions	

Part 2 (Continued)
Prenatal Visits

Monthly Visits 5th Month	Symptoms/Questions
Date	
Time A.M. P.M.	

Weight	Blood pressure

Changes from previous visit

Weight	Blood pressure

Diagnostic procedures

Special instructions

Monthly Visits 6th Month	Symptoms/Questions
Date	
Time A.M. P.M.	

Weight	Blood pressure

Changes from previous visit

Weight	Blood pressure

Diagnostic procedures

Special instructions

Part 2 (Continued)
Prenatal Visits

Monthly Visits 7th Month	Symptoms/Questions
Date	
Time A.M. P.M.	

Weight	Blood pressure
Changes from previous visit	
Weight	Blood pressure
Diagnostic procedures	

Special instructions

Monthly Visits 8th Month	Symptoms/Questions
Date	
Time A.M. P.M.	

Weight	Blood pressure
Changes from previous visit	
Weight	Blood pressure
Diagnostic procedures	

Special instructions

Part 2 (Continued)
Prenatal Visits

Monthly Visits 9th Month	Symptoms/Questions
Date	
Time A.M. P.M.	
Weight	Blood pressure
Changes from previous visit	
Weight	Blood pressure
Diagnostic procedures	
Special instructions	

Other Visits	Symptoms/Questions
Date	
Time A.M. P.M.	
Weight	Blood pressure
Changes from previous visit	
Weight	Blood pressure
Diagnostic procedures	
Special instructions	

Part 2 (Continued)
Prenatal Visits

Other Visits	Symptoms/Questions
Date	
Time A.M. P.M.	

Weight	Blood pressure
Changes from previous visit	
Weight	Blood pressure
Diagnostic procedures	

Special instructions

Other Visits	Symptoms/Questions
Date	
Time A.M. P.M.	

Weight	Blood pressure
Changes from previous visit	
Weight	Blood pressure
Diagnostic procedures	

Special instructions

PRENATAL VISITS RECORD

Part 3
Birth Summary

Name of child

Date of birth   Time of birth   A.M.   P.M.

Sex ☐ Female   ☐ Male

Weight   lbs   ozs   Length   inches

APGAR score   PKU test   Blood type

Place of birth   City   St

Facility/setting

Hospital

Address

Birthing center

Address

Other

Vaginal birth   ☐ Yes   ☐ No

C-section   ☐ Yes   ☐ No

Full term   ☐ Yes   ☐ No

If no, how many weeks premature

List any birthmark, birth defect, or complication noted at birth

Attending physician

Nurse-midwife

Other practitioner

Other information

PRESCRIPTION MEDICATIONS RECORD

Keeping track of your prescription medications is not only easy but it's also smart. The wise consumer always knows when a prescription was filled, the name of the medication (brand and generic), its expiration date, the prescribing physician's name, the pharmacy where it was filled, and any side effects or adverse reactions experienced. This Prescription Medications Record enables you to become a wise and informed consumer by putting essential information at your fingertips.

As you use this form, you'll realize the added benefit of assembling a medications profile. If you're taking more than one medication, there's always the risk of experiencing a drug interaction. By sharing your medications record with your practitioners, you can help them avoid prescribing medications that could cause you potentially serious health problems.

Enter the date you had the prescription filled in the first column on the form. Next, enter the name of the medication—either its brand or generic name. The brand name is the one given by the manufacturer to identify its particular medication and establish an identity separate from that of other manufacturers' products. The generic name is the actual chemical name of your medication and is often different from the brand name. Your pharmacist can give you these names.

The expiration date is very important because it can mean the difference between taking a product that is still effective or one that could do you harm. Manufacturers add an expiration date to medications to assure that a drug meets the standards established for it in terms of strength, quality, and purity when used before the date indicated. In addition to the manufacturer's expiration date, some states also mandate an expiration date (in some cases up to one year) from the date of dispensing. Expiration dates usually refer to medications that are in their original unopened containers and stored under proper conditions. Affixed to your prescription may be a warning label advising you not to use the medication beyond the date shown or different from the prescribed course of treatment as directed by your practitioner.

With more consumers doing comparison shopping to find the best price on medications, an accurate record of where you had your prescription filled is a must. Enter the name of the pharmacy, in the event that you have questions or want your prescription refilled at a later date. Especially critical is the documentation of any side effects or adverse reactions you experience while taking the drug. Some medications may cause unwanted side effects, such as headache or nausea, and others may cause life-threatening conditions, such as anaphylactic shock, impaired breathing, or irregular heartbeat. A word of warning: Adverse reactions usually necessitate your discontinuing the medication, and obviously some effects require medical attention. When you experience an unwanted effect, call your physician and pharmacist immediately.

PRESCRIPTION MEDICATIONS RECORD

List all prescription medications you have filled, including date filled, name of medication, expiration date, prescribing physician, pharmacy where filled, and any side effects (unwanted effects of the medication, such as dizziness, headache, or dry mouth) or adverse reactions (harmful, potentially life-threatening effects of the medication, such as anaphylactic shock, cardiac arrhythmia, or irregular breathing) you experience.

Date filled	Medication	Expiration date of medication	Prescribing physician	Pharmacy where filled	Side effects/Adverse reactions

PRESCRIPTION MEDICATIONS RECORD

Date filled	Medication	Expiration date of medication	Prescribing physician	Pharmacy where filled	Side effects/Adverse reactions

PRESCRIPTION MEDICATIONS RECORD

Date filled	Medication	Expiration date of medication	Prescribing physician	Pharmacy where filled	Side effects/Adverse reactions

PRESCRIPTION MEDICATIONS RECORD

Date filled	Medication	Expiration date of medication	Prescribing physician	Pharmacy where filled	Side effects/Adverse reactions

PRESCRIPTION MEDICATIONS RECORD

Date filled	Medication	Expiration date of medication	Prescribing physician	Pharmacy where filled	Side effects/Adverse reactions

PRESCRIPTION MEDICATIONS RECORD

Date filled	Medication	Expiration date of medication	Prescribing physician	Pharmacy where filled	Side effects/Adverse reactions

VISION CARE RECORD

Keeping an accurate record of visits to your eye care practitioners is easy with the Vision Care Record. Complete the questions in Part 1 relative to your current vision status and need for corrective lenses. Next, answer the questions concerning specific eye conditions you have or had. List the names, addresses, and telephone numbers of your vision practitioners, including ophthalmologists, optometrists, and opticians, in Part 2.

Use Part 3 every time you have an appointment with a practitioner. Keep all entries in chronological order—that way you can quickly locate the most up-to-date information about your eye health. Enter the practitioner's name and any symptoms or complaints you have. Use descriptive words, such as *dryness, itchiness, redness, tearing, puffiness, blurred vision*, and so on. Also indicate if one eye is affected more than the other. Your practitioner's examination will most likely include a check of your visual acuity (how well you see) at this time. Make sure you enter your visual acuity in the space provided for each eye. Remember, vision is expressed by two numbers, such as 20/20, 20/40, 20/100, and so on.

Enter the diagnosis made by your practitioner and any prescribed treatment or special instructions.

If you require corrective lenses, your practitioner will write a prescription for you. Be careful when recording this information since you don't want to accidently enter the wrong correction for each eye. Ask your practitioner for assistance if you're unsure as to how you should record the prescription, or—better yet—request a written copy of your lens prescription and attach it to this record.

VISION CARE RECORD

Complete the personal data and vision care history as requested in Part 1. In Part 2 list all current vision practitioners, including ophthalmologists, optometrists, and opticians. Use Part 3 to record any visits to your practitioners.

Part 1
Vision History

Do you wear glasses? Yes _____ No _____

If yes, are they single vision or bifocal lenses? Single _____ Bifocal _____

Age/year you began wearing glasses _____

Do you wear contact lenses? Yes _____ No _____

If yes, are they single vision or bifocal contacts? Single _____ Bifocal _____

Age/year you began wearing contact lenses _____

What type of contact lenses do you wear? Hard _____ Gas permeable _____

Soft _____ Daily wear _____ Extended wear _____ Reusable _____ Disposable _____

Do you have or have you had any of the following conditions? Indicate by check mark those conditions that apply and your age when the condition was diagnosed.

	Yes	No	Age		Yes	No	Age
Astigmatism				Injury to the eye			
Blepharitis (eyelid infection)				Loss of vision			
Cataract				Macular degeneration			
Color blindness				Posterior vitreous detachment			
Corneal abrasion							
Floaters				Retinal detachment			
Glaucoma							

Other vision problems not listed above

VISION CARE RECORD

Part 2
Vision Practitioners

Name
Specialty
Address   Suite
City   St   Zip   Telephone

Name
Specialty
Address   Suite
City   St   Zip   Telephone

Name
Specialty
Address   Suite
City   St   Zip   Telephone

Name
Specialty
Address   Suite
City   St   Zip   Telephone

Part 3
Individual Visits/Examinations Record

Date
Practitioner
Symptoms/Complaints/Treatments

Visual acuity   Right eye   /   Left eye   /
Prescription   Right eye +/-   Left eye +/-
Date of next appointment
Time   A.M.   P.M.

Part 3 (Continued)
Individual Visits/Examinations Record

Date

Practitioner

Symptoms/Complaints/Treatments

Visual acuity   Right eye   /   Left eye   /

Prescription   Right eye +/-   Left eye +/-

Date of next appointment

Time   A.M.   P.M.

Date

Practitioner

Symptoms/Complaints/Treatments

Visual acuity   Right eye   /   Left eye   /

Prescription   Right eye +/-   Left eye +/-

Date of next appointment

Time   A.M.   P.M.

Date

Practitioner

Symptoms/Complaints/Treatments

Visual acuity   Right eye   /   Left eye   /

Prescription   Right eye +/-   Left eye +/-

Date of next appointment

Time   A.M.   P.M.

Part 3 (Continued)
Individual Visits/Examinations Record

Date

Practitioner

Symptoms/Complaints/Treatments

Visual acuity   Right eye   /   Left eye   /

Prescription   Right eye +/-   Left eye +/-

Date of next appointment

Time   A.M.   P.M.

Date

Practitioner

Symptoms/Complaints/Treatments

Visual acuity   Right eye   /   Left eye   /

Prescription   Right eye +/-   Left eye +/-

Date of next appointment

Time   A.M.   P.M.

Date

Practitioner

Symptoms/Complaints/Treatments

Visual acuity   Right eye   /   Left eye   /

Prescription   Right eye +/-   Left eye +/-

Date of next appointment

Time   A.M.   P.M.

VISION CARE RECORD

Part 3 (Continued)
Individual Visits/Examinations Record

Date
Practitioner
Symptoms/Complaints/Treatments

Visual acuity   Right eye   /   Left eye   /
Prescription   Right eye +/-   Left eye +/-
Date of next appointment
Time   A.M.   P.M.

Date
Practitioner
Symptoms/Complaints/Treatments

Visual acuity   Right eye   /   Left eye   /
Prescription   Right eye +/-   Left eye +/-
Date of next appointment
Time   A.M.   P.M.

Date
Practitioner
Symptoms/Complaints/Treatments

Visual acuity   Right eye   /   Left eye   /
Prescription   Right eye +/-   Left eye +/-
Date of next appointment
Time   A.M.   P.M.

VISION CARE RECORD

Part 3 (Continued)
Individual Visits/Examinations Record

Date

Practitioner

Symptoms/Complaints/Treatments

Visual acuity   Right eye   /   Left eye   /

Prescription   Right eye +/-   Left eye +/-

Date of next appointment

Time   A.M.   P.M.

Date

Practitioner

Symptoms/Complaints/Treatments

Visual acuity   Right eye   /   Left eye   /

Prescription   Right eye +/-   Left eye +/-

Date of next appointment

Time   A.M.   P.M.

Date

Practitioner

Symptoms/Complaints/Treatments

Visual acuity   Right eye   /   Left eye   /

Prescription   Right eye +/-   Left eye +/-

Date of next appointment

Time   A.M.   P.M.

VISION CARE RECORD

Part 3 (Continued)
Individual Visits/Examinations Record

Date
Practitioner
Symptoms/Complaints/Treatments

Visual acuity   Right eye   /   Left eye   /
Prescription   Right eye +/-   Left eye +/-
Date of next appointment
Time   A.M.   P.M.

Date
Practitioner
Symptoms/Complaints/Treatments

Visual acuity   Right eye   /   Left eye   /
Prescription   Right eye +/-   Left eye +/-
Date of next appointment
Time   A.M.   P.M.

Date
Practitioner
Symptoms/Complaints/Treatments

Visual acuity   Right eye   /   Left eye   /
Prescription   Right eye +/-   Left eye +/-
Date of next appointment
Time   A.M.   P.M.

YOUR CHILD'S MEDICAL RECORD

This record asks you to begin a medical record for your child the day he or she is born. Why so soon? Obviously, as the primary advocate for your child's health, you are charged with the important task of keeping accurate and up-to-date medical information on him or her. A move from one community to another, a change of schools, or even a switch from one pediatric practitioner to another—in any of these situations and more, your ability to remain in control of the countless medical decisions to be made on behalf of your child is paramount. A good case can also be made for the value of these records to the child as he or she is an adult tracing current health problems to episodes of early childhood illness.

Start with day one. Enter the child's name, date of birth, time of birth, weight, length, APGAR score (results of a test that evaluates the general health of the newborn by examining the heart rate, respiratory effort, muscle tone, response to a tube in the nostril, and color), results of the PKU (phenylketonuria) test, and blood type.

Next, enter the place of birth, the facility (hospital, birthing center, home, or other), type of birth (vaginal or C-section), whether it was a full-term or premature delivery, and the name of the birth attendant. List any birthmarks, birth defects, or other complications.

Complete Part 2, Childhood Immunizations, by entering the name of the vaccine, date given, age of the child at the time, name of physician or nurse, and any side effects or adverse reactions observed. Use Part 3 to record all childhood illnesses, including date, condition and/or disease, age of child, physician, and treatment received.

Part 4 asks you to detail all periods of hospitalization, including the dates of admission and discharge, name of the hospital, reason for hospitalization, admitting physician, and any consulting physician(s).

YOUR CHILD'S MEDICAL RECORD

Part 1
Personal Data

Begin a medical record for each child by entering his or her personal data as requested. Use a separate page for each child.

Name of child

Date of birth   Time of birth   A.M.   P.M.

Sex   Female   Male   Weight   lbs   ozs   Length   inches

APGAR score   PKU test   Blood type

Place of birth   City   St

Facility/setting

Hospital

Address

Birthing center

Address

Other

Vaginal birth   Yes   No

C-section   Yes   No

Full term   Yes   No

If no, how many weeks premature

List any birthmark, birth defect, or complication noted at birth

Attending physician

Nurse-midwife

Other practitioner

Other information

Part 2
Childhood Immunizations

Enter the type of immunization, date, age of child, physician/nurse, and any side effects (unwanted effects, such as dizziness, headache, or dry mouth) or adverse reactions (harmful, potentially life-threatening effects such as anaphylactic shock, cardiac arrhythmia, or irregular breathing) your child experiences. Use this record for all immunizations from birth through adolescence and all other vaccinations that your child may receive.

Vaccine	Date	Age	Physician/ Nurse	Side effects or adverse reactions
Diphtheria, pertussis, tetanus (DPT)				
Oral polio				
Haemophilus influenzae type b (Hib)				
Hepatitis B (HBV)				
Measles, mumps, rubella (MMR)				
Tetanus and diphtheria (Td)				
Smallpox				

Part 3
Childhood Illnesses

Enter all periods of illness, including date, condition/disease, age of child, physician, and treatment received. Keep all entries in chronological order.

Date	Condition/ Disease	Child's Age	Physician	Treatment

Part 3 (Continued)
Childhood Illnesses

Date	Condition/ Disease	Child's Age	Physician	Treatment

Part 4
Childhood Hospitalizations

Enter all periods of hospitalization, including dates of admission and discharge, hospital, reason for hospitalization, admitting physician, and consulting physician(s).

Date Admitted	Discharged	Hospital	Reason for hospitalization	Physician(s) name(s)

YOUR CHILD'S MEDICAL RECORD

Part 1
Personal Data

Begin a medical record for each child by entering his or her personal data as requested. Use a separate page for each child.

Name of child

Date of birth _____ Time of birth ____ A.M. ____ P.M.

Sex ____ Female ____ Male ____ Weight ____ lbs ____ ozs Length ____ inches

APGAR score ____ PKU test ____ Blood type

Place of birth City _____ St

Facility/setting

Hospital

Address

Birthing center

Address

Other

Vaginal birth ____ Yes ____ No

C-section ____ Yes ____ No

Full term ____ Yes ____ No

If no, how many weeks premature

List any birthmark, birth defect, or complication noted at birth

_____

_____

_____

Attending physician

Nurse-midwife

Other practitioner

_____

_____

Other information

_____

_____

_____

_____

_____

_____

_____

_____

YOUR CHILD'S MEDICAL RECORD

Part 2
Childhood Immunizations

Enter the type of immunization, date, age of child, physician/nurse, and any side effects (unwanted effects, such as dizziness, headache, or dry mouth) or adverse reactions (harmful, potentially life-threatening effects such as anaphylactic shock, cardiac arrhythmia, or irregular breathing) your child experiences. Use this record for all immunizations from birth through adolescence and all other vaccinations that your child may receive.

Vaccine	Date	Age	Physician/Nurse	Side effects or adverse reactions
Diphtheria, pertussis, tetanus (DPT)				
Oral polio				
Haemophilus influenzae type b (Hib)				
Hepatitis B (HBV)				
Measles, mumps, rubella (MMR)				
Tetanus and diphtheria (Td)				
Smallpox				

Part 3
Childhood Illnesses

Enter all periods of illness, including date, condition/disease, age of child, physician, and treatment received. Keep all entries in chronological order.

Date	Condition/ Disease	Child's Age	Physician	Treatment

Part 3 (Continued)
Childhood Illnesses

Date	Condition/ Disease	Child's Age	Physician	Treatment

Part 4
Childhood Hospitalizations

Enter all periods of hospitalization, including dates of admission and discharge, hospital, reason for hospitalization, admitting physician, and consulting physician(s).

Date Admitted	Discharged	Hospital	Reason for hospitalization	Physician(s) name(s)